BODY
CONFIDENT

BODY CONFIDENT

Unlock the secret to strength, independence, and lifelong badassery using the F2 Method

Bronson Dant

Body Confident copyright © 2024 by Bronson Dant
Coach Bronson
Reston, VA 20190
coachbronson.com
Send feedback to bronson@coachbronson.com

Publisher's Cataloging-in-Publication

Names: Dant, Bronson, author.
Title: Body Confident: Unlock the secret to strength, independence, and lifelong badassery using the F2 Method / Bronson Dant.
Description: Reston, VA : BD Solutions, [2024] | Includes bibliographical references.
Identifiers: ISBN: 979-8-9901241-1-0 (hardcover) | 979-8-9901241-0-3 (softcover) | 979-8-9901241-2-7 (ebook) | 979-8-9901241-3-4 (audiobook)
Subjects: LCSH: Physical fitness--Psychological aspects. | Self-confidence. | Body image. | Health. | LCGFT: Self-help publications.
Classification: LCC: GV481.2 .D37 2024 | DDC: 613.7--dc23

Special discounts for bulk sales are available.
Please contact bronson@apxts.com.

Thank you to my Muse.

Contents

Tell Me What You Think

Let other readers know what you thought of *Body Confident*. Please write an honest review for this book on your favorite online bookshop.

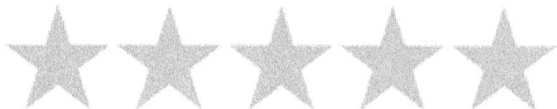

★ ★ ★ ★ ★

FOREWORD BY DR. PHILIP OVADIA

As a cardiothoracic surgeon, I have seen firsthand the devastating effects of poor health on the human body. It's a problem compounded by the overwhelming amount of conflicting information on health and fitness that exists today. People are bombarded with various diets, exercise routines, and health advice, often leading to confusion and frustration. This is why I am excited to write this foreword for *Body Confident* by Bronson Dant, a book that serves as a practical guide to navigating the complexities of health and fitness.

Bronson's F2 Method, outlined in this book, is a testament to the power of individualized approaches to health. It's not about following a one-size-fits-all plan but about finding what works for you. This book is a critical thinking tool for your health journey, empowering you to make informed decisions based on your unique needs and goals.

I am particularly impressed by the practicality of the information presented in *Body Confident*. It's not just theoretical; it's actionable. The five core concepts of the F2 Method provide a solid foundation for anyone looking to improve their health and fitness. This book is a valuable resource for anyone seeking to take control of their health, cut through the noise of conflicting advice, and find a sustainable path to wellness.

I am deeply honored to be part of this message and to help bring this important information to those who need it most. It's time for people to become confident in their bodies and their health, and *Body Confident* is a crucial step in that direction. I commend Bronson for his dedication to helping others achieve their health and fitness goals, and I am confident that this book will significantly impact the lives of its readers.

- Dr. Philip Ovadia, Author of *Stay off My Operating Table*

"Body Confidence is the freedom to engage in life to its fullest because you trust your body to perform and protect you."
- Coach Bronson

PREFACE

In 2022 I wanted to take the concepts I was using with my clients and document what happened when they were applied consistently for eight weeks. I had been running fitness and nutrition challenges for a few years and, after selling my gym, had moved to a completely virtual version of the program. The idea was to find out exactly how effective a program, built on the concepts you're about to learn about, could be for women over forty-five dealing with the symptoms and effects of menopause.

There was no focus on fat loss, blood markers, mitochondria, or any specific mechanism of biology. No biohacks or overly complicated protocols, products, or supplements were used when applying the F2 Method in this challenge. It was a simple program designed to meet the basic needs of each woman's mindset, fitness, and nutrition. The program utilized concepts of the F2 Method and met each woman exactly where they were. The results and details of the peer-reviewed, eight-week case study, titled *Changes in body composition and physical performance in peri and post-menopausal women following a ketogenic diet and functional fitness program*, were published in the IP Journal of Nutrition, Metabolism and Health Science in Sept of 2022. (https://www.jnmhs.com/article-details/17344)

What you'll find in the case study validates the effectiveness of the F2 Method and shows how individuals can duplicate the process. The F2 Method, when applied properly, can be replicated and scaled to anyone's current situation, goals, or timeline.

Besides having results like increasing Skeletal Muscle Mass Percentage and decreasing Body Fat Percentage, study participants reported improvements in several aspects of health and fitness, directly impacting the quality of life. Some of the improvements were:

- Strength
- Endurance

- Stamina
- Flexibility
- Energy
- Blood Pressure
- Sleep
- Resting Heart Rate
- Body Measurements
- Inflammation
- Satiety

The feedback from the participants was overwhelmingly positive about how the program improved their quality of life. The improvements seen in body composition and demonstrated by the fitness benchmarks provide indicators that explain the connection between physical ability and an individual's quality of life. Here are a few comments from participants:

> *"I lost body fat and weight and gained skeletal muscle mass which is what I wanted to do. I am stronger, my stamina is better, and I can do more standard push-ups than I ever had before. The progress I got from the challenge is more than I expected I would get, and I am extremely happy about it."*
>
> *"My biggest takeaway was that I can do more than I thought I could do and that my only limitations are the ones I put on myself."*
>
> *"It's not really a challenge. It's learning about your body physically and mentally. Each participant has different needs. We all come together to encourage and share our struggles and our triumphs. Our coach sets the foundation and guides us to make it our own."*

The path forward is understanding the importance of mindset, fitness, and nutrition. If you look beyond meal plans and strict workout routines and practice the principles of the F2 Method, you will have greater success in achieving body confidence and improving your quality of life.

INTRODUCTION

A re you confident in your body? Do you have any idea what that feels like?

How different would your life be if you never worried about what your body could do? How freely could you live, if your physical ability was never in question? Do you struggle with being self-conscious about how you look? Do you wonder what it's like when you see a fit athletic person walk into a room and everyone looks at them with respect? Does your lack of confidence in your appearance affect your mood, or how you relate to people? Are you tired of being sick or hurt all the time?

Body confidence is having zero doubt that you can handle any situation. It's knowing that your body is functioning properly and can perform any task you need it to. Body confidence is having pride in the work and consistent effort you've put in to keep yourself at the top of your game.

Words used to define "confident;" sure, certain, positive, self-assured, self-reliant, bold, intrepid, and unperturbed. How often do you feel these things about yourself?

In order to be Body Confident, you have to optimize and improve your quality of life. I'll discuss this more further in the book, but understand that your journey is not about weight loss or flat abs. Once you understand this, you'll understand why everything you've been doing hasn't worked as well or lasted as long as you'd like it to.

You dutifully bought gym equipment, participated in fitness challenges, tried supplements, and tracked calories, macros, and reps. Drinking smoothies, eating salads, running 5Ks, and monitoring your water intake is routine. However, looking in the mirror, your reflection ponders why all the pushups, cardio, and macros fail to move the needle. When you see bouts of progress, why do you yo-yo on the scale and then bounce to the next fad diet?

There is more information available on health and fitness now than there has ever been. This access to information is simultaneously a massive blessing and a terrible curse. Something you watch or read may sound like the perfect solution when in reality, it has nothing to do with your situation or goals. This disconnect is why those claims of eating sticks of butter for weight loss work for a few, but not you.

It's like you are stuck in the weeds of too much *specific* information.

As impressive as the Internet is, knowledge without context and understanding creates more problems than it fixes. Fad diets, harmful exercise routines, and often unnecessary supplements will leave your head spinning. You know what I am talking about. Sardine fasts, priming and fasting, chugging power supplements, dips, sit-ups, and lunges galore. Can these things work? Sure, but how long will you throw stuff at the wall and hope it sticks?

Over the last decade or so, my job as a coach has been to help people pull themselves out of the weeds and make progress by stepping back a bit, understanding the principles that get results, and applying them to individual contexts. Optimal health and quality of life are not exclusively about fat loss and exercise. So, this book is not about how to lose weight or get six-pack abs. This book is about helping you improve your quality of life, increase physical independence, and be the best version of yourself. I believe that health, fitness, and wellness are interconnected and that one cannot be achieved without the others.

The F2 Method is a way of understanding the inter-relationship of each aspect of health and how those relationships impact your quality of life. We tend to isolate and compartmentalize concepts and ideas to suit our needs, which often leads to a lack of comprehension about how those concepts work together. The F2 Method makes those connections and helps you apply them.

First, we have to understand that historically Western medicine views optimal health and wellness from a single point—symptoms. If you treat the symptoms, you will be healthy. Address the pain, discomfort, or irregular test result, and poof, you are better. However, when we treat the symptom, we fail to address the root cause. The F2 Method will help you discover that optimal health is based on five core concepts. Optimal Health is:

- Unique to every individual.
- Comprehensive, not just symptom-focused.
- Concept based. There are no hard and fast rules, only guidelines.
- Should be sustainable. Fad diets and excessive exercise are not sustainable.
- Measurable through meeting realistic and individualized goals.

From here, you will learn that you gain a healthy quality of life by focusing on the trifecta of mindset, fitness, and nutrition. Like a three-legged stool, your health cannot stand or be stable if one leg is missing. Further, each leg must be strong enough to support the weight it bears. Thus, each leg has a foundation in three of the nine tenets. All perfectly balanced. Together, they support optimal health and healthy quality of life.

Now, you may wonder why you should listen to me. After all, I am just another fitness coach claiming to have the magic potion. To that, I would say—yes, I am a fitness coach. However, my passion for what I do is deeply personal. I've been there. Reflections in the mirror or unsolicited photographs caught me off guard and had me asking if that person was really me. I was overweight, tired, and frustrated. Like many others, I tried everything only to fall back off the wagon, put weight back on, and feel like everything I had done was for naught. I lacked body confidence and it was a miserable way to live.

I want to share my story and method because I know it works. I know it works from a personal perspective. The F2 Method works for my clients and can work for you. Using the F2 Method in your journey to better health will be your guide to success.

This is where body confidence comes into play. Body confidence, as I define it, is not just about looking good. It's about knowing and trusting in the capabilities and resilience of your body because of the time and effort you've invested in building your physical ability and metabolic function. It's about feeling secure and competent in any environment, proud of your health, and strength.

Body confidence means understanding that you are in control of your body and your health, and that's a power no one can take from you.

Are you with me? Let's start with important foundational knowledge and explore why some things work for certain people and not for others. I will share my personal story of struggling with health. You will learn why your individuality is crucial on this journey and discover what metabolism is and is not. We'll dive into the F2 Method. You will learn core concepts and the guiding tenets that make the process easy to follow. Finally, we'll go over some things you can do on your own to implement and practice the F2 Method and achieve body confidence.

Let's get it!

CHAPTER 1

- -

YOU'RE NOT ALONE

"The real voyage of discovery consists not in seeking new landscapes, but in having new eyes."
~ Marcel Proust

Humans have an innate fear of change. We will only embrace it when we fear our current circumstances more than the unknown that comes with change. A realization often ignites fear, and we decide to do something different. We tell ourselves *something's gotta change.* I know because I've been there.

I was overweight, uncomfortable, anxious, and out of shape. I was making good money, had a good life, and wasn't paying any attention to what was happening in my body. I was content and in denial about where my health and quality of life were.

In my late thirties, I was over 240 pounds. I had man boobs, acne, and irritable bowels, which led to urgent bowels and high levels of anxiety. I went to the gym regularly to check the box, but it was more of a social event than an intentional effort at self-improvement.

I had zero body confidence.

One summer, I took my kids to the beach. My daughter took a picture of me sitting in a chair by the water. This moment was a rare occurrence because, at the time, I rarely let people take photos of me. Isn't it funny how we can be *okay* where we are, but deep down, we know things aren't right, and we don't want any part of something that makes us face the facts?

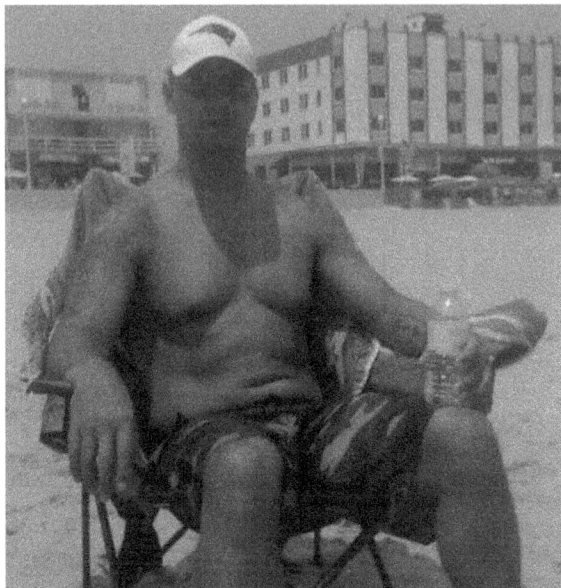

When I saw that picture, I knew something had to change. I could no longer exist in the reality I had created.

I had convinced myself that I was still the gung-ho kid who never had to worry about what he ate, joined the Army, and stayed fit by being active and working hard.

Obviously, that all stopped being true fifteen years prior. I was almost forty, sat at a desk all day, and rarely broke a sweat. I regularly ate copious amounts of French fries, pizza, ice cream, spoons of sugar with some coffee added, and every kind of noodle I could get my hands on.

With this image etched into my mind, I had a choice to make. I could either accept my current reality or create a new one. I decided to create a new one. I had no idea what I was in for.

I knew I needed to change how I ate. I also knew that my fitness routine wouldn't get the job done. I didn't have a specific goal at that point; I just didn't want to see what I saw in the mirror anymore. I started looking for a fitness program to follow and made one significant change in my diet. I stopped eating French fries!

French Fries

The amount of French fries I ate in a week was excessive, to say the least. At this time in my life, I worked in IT, and at least three days a week, I would go with friends to Red Robin for lunch. If you're familiar with Red Robin, you know they have many burger options and bottomless French fries. Yup, not just a side of fries added to a plate; they give you as many baskets as you want!

Each time I would go there for lunch, I would get a chili burger with bacon, and I would not leave until I had eaten at least two baskets of fries. My thought process was if I'm paying for bottomless fries, I'm getting my money's worth. The sad part about this story is that Red Robin French fries were only a fraction of my fry problem.

McDonald's, Mission BBQ, Boardwalk Fries, and any restaurant that served fries, tater tots, or hash browns was unsafe from my addiction to fried potatoes! During this time, I never had less than five days a week without eating some sort of fried food. It was the big elephant in the room that I knew I had to focus on.

Did I go cold turkey? Heck no. I started by making a simple but difficult change. I stopped eating out as much. I knew I wouldn't have as much access or exposure to French fries if I made my own food. So, I started food prepping, bringing my lunch to work, and going out for dinner a little less. That helped a lot. It took time, but eventually became part of my routine. It didn't get me all the way though.

The next thing I did was commit that when I did go out, I would not get fries with any of my meals. I began to practice controlling my environment and asking for what I needed. Did it work all the time? Nope. Sometimes the food would come with fries, and I would eat them; sometimes, I wouldn't. But I kept asking myself if fries were really helping me get where I wanted to go.

It took more than a year for me to get to a place where I could see French fries and not have an automatic impulse to grab one and eat it. It's been over ten years since I've had French fries more than once a year. Do I enjoy them? Absolutely! Do I need them like I used to? Absolutely not.

French fries were only one of many foods I needed to break from, and it's taken me several years to work through all of them. I won't get into the amount of Ben & Jerry's I used to eat, the large meat lover's pizzas I'd eat in one sitting, or the giant double orders of Pad Thai with double spring rolls that made up my dinner multiple times a week.

The biggest lesson French fries taught me was how to take small steps and build a habit of change. The power that the concept of habit change has is significant. If you learn it in one area, you've learned it in all areas of your life. If I can break myself from my numerous attachments to these foods, you can too.

Do You Even Lift, Bro?

My fitness journey started, like most people, with Google. I looked up all sorts of workout programs I could do to get in shape with my membership at Planet Fitness. I tried different things occasionally and even signed up for a twelve-week online program with daily workouts, accountability, nutrition, coaching, and all the bells and whistles. None of it stuck. I wasn't consistent. I felt lost and completely out of my depth.

Then Dominick Maurici came into my life and changed everything. Dominick is the owner of Caution CrossFit in Miami, Florida. Just before I turned forty, I went on a cruise to celebrate, where I met Dominick. More accurately, that's where I saw him throwing around eighty-pound dumbbells like they were paperweights!

There I was on the elliptical; there he was doing actual fitness. I had to approach him and ask him what he was doing. It looked cool as hell. Thankfully, Dominick is a great guy and answered my questions. The rest of the week, we hung out and worked out together. Dominick was patient and didn't push me to do what he was doing. He demonstrated what it means to meet someone where they are. He showed me more about CrossFit and opened my eyes to what fitness could be.

When I got home from the cruise, I canceled the program I was in and immediately found a CrossFit gym to join. That was the beginning of the incredible journey I've been on over the last decade. CrossFit is where everything came together for me. It didn't happen all at once, but the foundation for my understanding of fitness and how tightly all the other aspects of health are intertwined started there.

CrossFit taught me that everyone is different, but the principles of movement apply to everyone. One of the best quotes from Greg Glassman, the founder of CrossFit, is, "The needs of the elderly and professional athletes differ by degree, not kind." I learned many of the fitness concepts and principles in this book from my training and experience as a Certified CrossFit Trainer and owning a CrossFit gym for over five years.

The other thing that CrossFit did for me was open an entire world of possibilities for how I could progress and grow. Until CrossFit, my only goal was to *get jacked* or *ripped*. With CrossFit, I learned there were hundreds of different things I could get my body to do that had no relationship with my weight or appearance. I started setting goals that immediately impacted my physical ability and freed me from anxiety over what my body could or couldn't do.

Since I got my first CrossFit certification, I have accumulated practical, hands-on experience working with hundreds of people from all walks of life. I realized that what I was helping people with, had less to do with weight loss and more with the quality of life. This realization grew as I learned and worked with more people year after year. It wasn't until I took a leap and tried a crazy nutrition idea that everything fell into place.

Back and Forth

Before I get into the crazy nutrition plan I started, I want to talk about the improvement process and the frustration that can come with it. I went through a lot of ups and downs in my journey to get healthy and gain back the body confidence I had when I was younger. From where I started, you can see that making fundamental changes to my diet and getting into a solid fitness program made a big difference. I was in great shape!

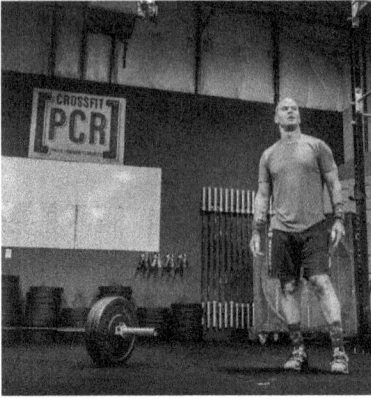

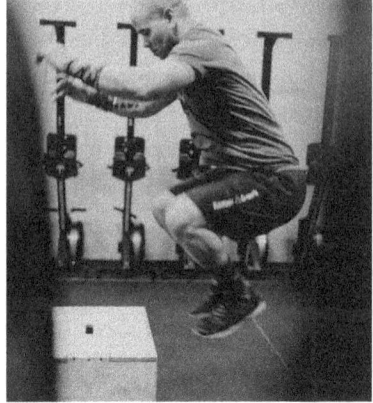

This was progress. I had improved my physical ability and even changed my body composition dramatically. Adding fitness to my life helped me lose about forty pounds, improve my strength, and reinforce my desire to maintain a healthy lifestyle. But it wasn't enough.

Like many people, I was doing a lot of work to stay in shape. The problem was, no matter how hard I worked, I could only get so far. My weight hit a wall. I stopped progressing in my fitness because the more I worked, the more I hurt. My recovery only got worse, and the injuries started piling up.

Over the span of a few years, I had two torn calves, multiple pulled hamstrings, a strained adductor, torn labrums in both shoulders, and a torn meniscus in my left knee. On top of that, I had to work out less and less each week because I always felt beat down. It would be a good week if I could get three workouts in without falling apart.

After a couple of years of this, most of the improvements I had seen in my body composition and fitness started to erode. By the time I was in my mid-forties, I had put back on thirty pounds and felt horrible about my progress or lack of it. As a gym owner and someone responsible for teaching and guiding people to a better quality of life, I needed to find an answer to what was happening.

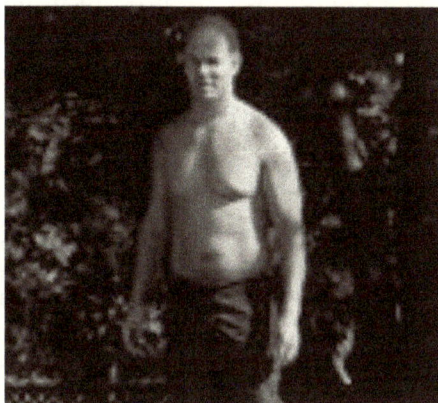

Going through this process helped me realize that no matter how hard you work, you can never complete the puzzle if you're not looking at the whole picture. Effort alone will only get you so far. You need to have a direction and a plan that addresses every aspect of the things impacting your life. I started to understand how we are more than what we eat, what we do, or what we think; we are all of them combined. This realization led me to stop eating vegetables and experiment with the carnivore diet.

I know what you are thinking—*another fad diet*. But hear me out. It's not about the specific diet. It is about what works for you and following guidelines, not rules.

Releasing the Carnivore

Fitness, by itself, wasn't working. I needed to do something different. When I first heard about the carnivore diet, I was already following a very clean, Paleo diet. It was moderate in protein and fat with reasonably *healthy* carb sources like sweet potatoes, rice, and lots of leafy greens and other veggies.

I figured I was eating as clean as possible and working out as well as I could imagine, so something must not be optimal for me to still have urgent bowels, body composition issues, poor recovery, numerous injuries, and feeling horrible in my body overall.

Over the years, I had tried low-fat diets, Whole 30, sugar detoxes, and other diet protocols. All the time, I was focusing on moderation and decreasing processed foods. At least I knew processed food was not the best. Still, nothing was changing. Then I was introduced to the idea of not eating vegetables.

What?!?!

A Licensed Dietitian Nutritionist (LDN) told me about the concept and recommended I look into it to help with my recovery and as an elimination diet to see if my urgent bowel symptoms would improve. The idea was to try it for sixty to ninety days and see what happened.

I did some research and found out there were more people than I ever expected who had been eating zero veggies for years. Did I wonder about Vitamin C, where I'd get all my nutrients from, what would happen to my cholesterol and all those things? Absolutely. But I had already tried so many things. I figured what could a couple of months do that would be so bad. I could always take extra vitamins or supplements if I needed to. So, I decided to try it. That was over five years ago!

I went all in from day one. I ate what I had in the house and kept going. I didn't know I was in for one surprise after another. I was unprepared for how tremendous this change was in my life. Sixty to ninety days came and went.

Over five years later, my quality of life and my passion for living it have exploded in a way that is hard to describe. I am over fifty years old and I feel like I'm a teenager again. The energy, excitement, and potential I've created for myself are mind-boggling.

I first noticed that I wasn't as hungry throughout the day. I ate two times a day and started thinking about food less. My snacking between meals slowed to a crawl, then stopped altogether.

Then I noticed that while my workouts were not the best, I felt better after them. I had low energy for several weeks as my body adapted, but I slowly increased my workout frequency without feeling so rundown and worn out.

Within a few months, I saw significant strength gains and dramatic improvement in my conditioning and high-intensity workouts. There was a period when I set a personal record (PR) in some aspect of fitness every single workout. It was insane!

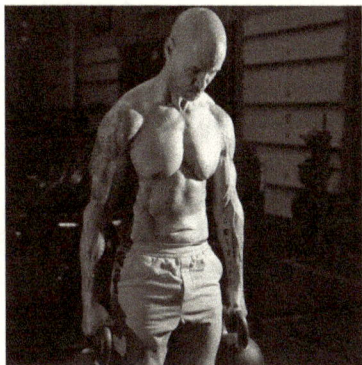

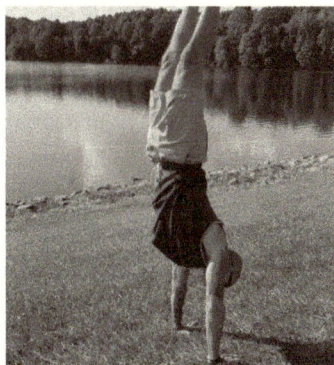

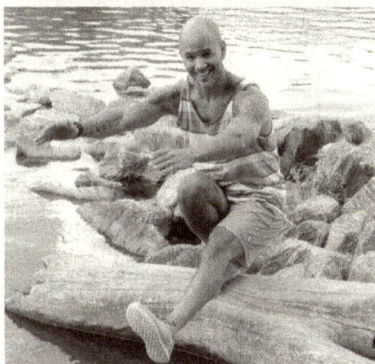

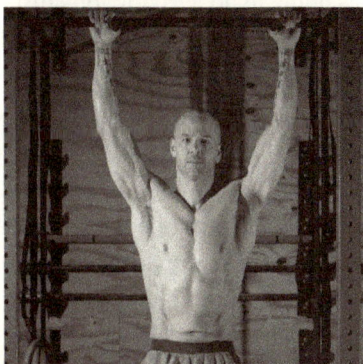

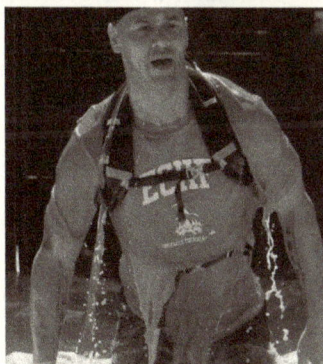

Changing to the carnivore diet tremendously impacted my physical fitness and body composition and made my lifestyle easier to manage. Food prep and shopping are magnitudes easier when all you're preparing is meat and eggs. I saw the most significant benefits from cutting out veggies in my overall health.

My urgent bowels and the commensurate issues that come with it were legendary, and not in a good way. It was standard practice for everyone I knew to avoid being in enclosed spaces or stuck in any periods of extended travel with me. My ability to identify, locate, or access bathroom facilities was the leading factor in every decision I made in just about every situation.

I couldn't get in a car without going to the bathroom. When I arrived, I had to know where the bathroom was. I often had to interrupt whatever I was doing to go. Driving long distances, flying, and even getting on a bus was utterly nerve-racking because I never knew when I would need to go or if I would have a place to go.

I have been stuck in traffic and crapped my pants. I used to keep toilet paper or paper towels in my trunk so that if I needed to stop on the side of the road at any time, I was prepared. I refilled my trunk several times over the years. Embarrassingly, I have had to do my business on the side of the road in multiple states and countries.

It's hard to explain how much anxiety and stress I lived with every day. I had been dealing with these things for so long that I didn't even realize how bad it had gotten until it was gone. About ninety days into carnivore, I realized I hadn't had to rush to the bathroom in weeks. I realized that the things I was doing to prepare for the inevitable were wasted because the unavoidable wasn't happening.

It took less than three months for the complete removal of vegetables to totally eliminate any urgent bowel issues I had. It's been over five years since. I may not have lost 150 pounds, but I now feel more free and relaxed about my life than I ever could have before.

You may be thinking, *great, now he's trying to sell me on the carnivore diet*. Nothing could be further from the truth. I share my story of the carnivore experience to highlight that I was following what Western medicine recommended, which wasn't working. One of the three legs of the stool was unstable. I had to break from what I thought worked for everyone else and create an individualized plan. This book is not about selling you on a specific diet but helping you explore the ideas about why things work, not how they work. Here's what I mean. The carnivore diet is effective because it increases nutrient density, bioavailability, and satiety. That's *why* it works. That's what it does for you. Eating mainly animal meat provides increased consumption of animal protein and saturated fats, which stimulate metabolic hormone production, improve digestive enzymatic function, and trigger satiety hormone secretion. That's *how* it works.

You don't need to know how it works to understand what it does for your progress.

At fifty-one, the last five years of my life have been the most productive, exciting, and passionate. I have learned to combine the principles of fitness and nutrition with my experience as a coach helping hundreds of people fix their mindset and stop limiting their progress. The F2 Method is what got me to where I am today. It's what I use every single day to help people get where they want to be.

My story isn't that different from many people's. We are not alone. Everyone has similar struggles and challenges. If you think there is a way and have a method for navigating through those challenges, you can never be stopped. What we must remember is wellness lives on a continuum.

Takeaways

- Change only happens when your pain or discomfort becomes greater than the pain or discomfort of the change itself.
- Start with the thing that will make the biggest impact. It can be a small change. It doesn't have to be a large sweeping overhaul of your life.
- Stacking success over time will lead to sustained progress.
- Your journey will not happen in a straight line.
- You have to be willing to try new things that may go against popular opinion or "known" science.

Resources

- Get **FREE** Bonus material that includes a complete breakdown and analysis of the most common fitness and nutrition programs to help you evaluate which ones will work best for you by following the F2 Method.
- Join **Coach Bronson's Body Confident Support Group** on Discord and meet more people who are improving themselves every day. https://discord.coachbronson.com
- Download the **FREE Body Confident Book Bonus Material** and Community information at https://bodyconfidentbook.com.

CHAPTER 2

- -

ADDRESSING THE INDIVIDUAL

*"You must go on adventures alone to find out where
you belong."~ Sue Fitzmaurice*

The F2 Method is a process that puts *you* at the center of improving your quality of life. It's all about evaluating information, making choices, and measuring results. The individual is the basis for every decision, the implementer of each action, and the focal point of all results.

The individual is you.

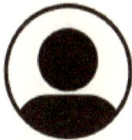 **The Individual**

Everyone is unique, so what works for your best friend may not work for you, just as the classic diets didn't work for me. Understanding the individual factors that determine your health and quality of life is very important. Let's examine wellness and how you define it for yourself.

The Wellness Continuum

Quality of life should be defined for lifestyle decisions to have value. Experience shows that the definition of quality of life must include physical and mental or emotional health because these aspects are closely intertwined, and both significantly impact your overall well-being.

All too often, the focus is placed on pain, discomfort, or dissatisfaction in a person's life without understanding the broader impact other environmental or lifestyle habits have on that specific thing.

Understanding the Wellness Continuum offers a comprehensive perspective, demonstrating that health, fitness, and wellness are not isolated concepts. Instead, they are interrelated facets of a broader picture. By adopting the Wellness Continuum as a guiding paradigm, you can recognize the interconnectedness of all fitness, health, and wellness aspects.

The **number one concept** you need to understand is that all health measures are the same, no matter what you're referencing.

No matter how you measure Fitness, Health, or Wellness—you're measuring the same thing.

Weakness, immobility, injury, metabolic syndrome, insulin resistance, and depression are all on one side of the quality of life spectrum. Strength, resilience, metabolic flexibility, and cognitive ability are on the other side. The factors involved in all of them are intertwined and inseparable.

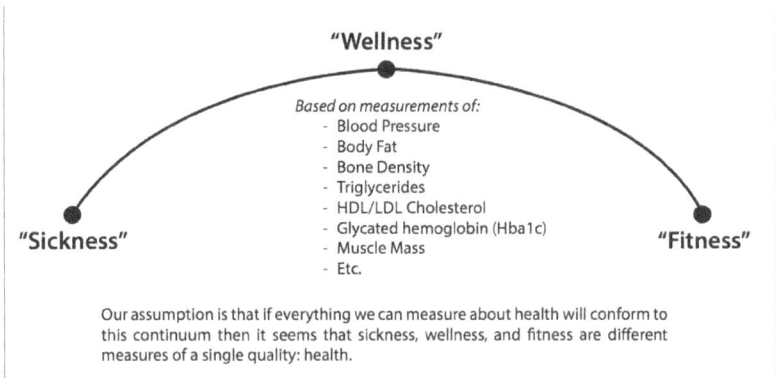

"Wellness"

Based on measurements of:
- Blood Pressure
- Body Fat
- Bone Density
- Triglycerides
- HDL/LDL Cholesterol
- Glycated hemoglobin (Hba1c)
- Muscle Mass
- Etc.

"Sickness"   **"Fitness"**

Our assumption is that if everything we can measure about health will conform to this continuum then it seems that sickness, wellness, and fitness are different measures of a single quality: health.

Image 1 - Wellness Continuum

Visualize the Wellness Continuum as a sliding scale that runs from sickness to optimal wellness. When you isolate and treat aspects of your health individually, you ignore this continuum. Doing so leads to short-term solutions and often fails to address the root causes of your issues. It's like placing a band-aid over a wound that requires surgery. The band-aid might stop the bleeding temporarily, but it does not address the underlying problem.

In contrast, when you understand the Wellness Continuum, your efforts to improve one aspect of your well-being can have positive ripple effects across the entire health spectrum. For example, a commitment to regular physical exercise can enhance your physical fitness and directly improve your health by reducing the risk of many diseases. But the benefits don't stop there. Regular exercise can also boost mental and emotional wellness by reducing stress, anxiety, and depression symptoms and improving mood and overall cognitive function.

Understanding the Wellness Continuum and the relationships between health, fitness, and wellness allows you to make informed decisions that positively impact your entire well-being. This knowledge helps you move from a state of mere survival into a state of optimal thriving.

The F2 Method emphasizes this integrated view of health and wellness. It does not seek just to eliminate illness or enhance fitness. Instead, it aims for holistic wellness. The goal is to enable you to function at your absolute best in every area of your life.

The importance of the Wellness Continuum underscores the value of prevention. Instead of waiting for illness to strike and then reacting, you can proactively work toward wellness, building resilience against potential health issues in the future. Don't just aim to add years to your life, but also life to your years.

The Wellness Continuum is an essential paradigm that guides an understanding of health, fitness, and wellness. It reminds you that every aspect of life is interconnected. Every choice can move you closer to wellness or push you toward illness. By embracing the F2 Method and the Wellness Continuum, you can make choices that enhance your overall quality of life and set you on the path to becoming the *best version of yourself*.

Changing how you view wellness is a big first step to freeing yourself from the mental limitations keeping you locked into an on-again, off-again cycle of success and failure. Are you ready for another topic you can learn to look at differently? Let's talk about metabolism and walk through how your metabolism isn't slow or fast and how it really works.

Systems of Function: Understanding Your Metabolism

No, metabolism is not how you burn calories. Metabolism is the chemical process that converts food to energy. We believe we are healthier or skinnier when we think of *high metabolism*. However, metabolism will naturally regulate to meet our individual needs. Metabolism is rarely the cause of how much you weigh, the weight you lose, or how much you gain. Studies have even shown that overweight people often have a fast metabolism. The reason is they require more energy for essential body functions. Their basal metabolic rate (BMR) is higher to meet their functional needs.

Your BMR refers to how many calories your body needs to function while at rest, and, like everything else we have discussed, your BMR will vary. Your age, sex, muscle mass, genes, and other factors like caloric intake can affect your BMR. Now, I know I said this isn't about how you burn calories. However, I have to address the elephant in the room for those who want to insist that a reduction in calories will help with weight loss.

Don't skip meals or restrict calories, hoping you will *improve your metabolism*. When you skip meals or restrict calories, you will force your metabolism to adapt. It will use fewer calories and eat away your body mass for energy. With that, let's talk about what metabolism really means.

When you exercise or change your diet, you tend to think of the benefits you can see and feel, like increased strength, improved endurance, less inflammation, more energy, less brain fog, and so on. But the truth is, the benefits of enhancing your lifestyle go much deeper than just the physical changes you can see and feel. In fact, when you work to improve your lifestyle, you are actually improving your body's three major Systems of Function:

- **Biology**: The complex interactions and processes carried out by cells, tissues, and organs to maintain life, including growth, reproduction, response to stimuli, and homeostasis.
- **Physiology**: How the systems and organs operate and interact to perform vital activities, such as respiration, digestion, circulation, and regulation of temperature.
- **Neurology**: The activities of the brain, spinal cord, and nerves, including the processing of sensory information, coordination of movement, and regulation of cognitive and emotional responses.

All three Systems of Function ARE your *metabolism*.

Biology

Metabolism is your biology. Biology encompasses the fundamental processes that form the foundation of living organisms, including humans. You can stimulate positive biological changes in your body through exercise and proper nutrition. Regular exercise has been shown to reduce the risk of chronic diseases, such as heart disease, diabetes, and certain cancers, while also improving immune function, helping you combat illness and disease more effectively. You support your overall biological health and well-being by engaging in physical activity and adopting a nutritious diet.

Exercise also plays a significant role in supporting immune function. Moderate-intensity physical activity has been shown to boost the production of immune cells, improve immune surveillance, and enhance the body's ability to fight off infections and diseases. Additionally, regular exercise has been associated with a reduced risk of upper respiratory tract infections and a faster recovery from illness.

In conjunction with exercise, proper nutrition is vital for supporting our biological processes. A diet that includes an adequate intake of essential macronutrients (protein and fats) and essential vitamins and minerals provides the necessary building blocks for the body to function optimally. Protein, in particular, is crucial for tissue repair, growth, and maintenance. It supports the development of lean muscle mass, aids post-exercise recovery, and helps regulate metabolic processes.

Consuming a nutrient-rich diet supports cellular function, promotes proper digestion and nutrient absorption, and contributes to overall health and vitality.

By incorporating regular exercise and proper nutrition into our lifestyles, we can harness the power of biology to enhance our health, reduce the risk of diseases, and improve overall well-being. The human body consists of numerous biological processes that occur to maintain its normal function. Here is a list of some major biological processes that occur in the human body:

- **Cell division:** Cells in the body undergo division through processes like mitosis and meiosis, leading to growth, tissue repair, and reproduction.
- **DNA replication:** DNA molecules are replicated during the cell division to ensure genetic continuity and transmission of genetic information.
- **Protein synthesis:** Cells synthesize proteins through transcription and translation, essential for various functions such as enzyme activity, structural support, and cell signaling.
- **DNA transcription and translation:** DNA is transcribed into messenger RNA (mRNA), then translated into proteins by ribosomes.
- **Immune response:** The immune system defends the body against pathogens and foreign substances through phagocytosis, antibody production, and cell-mediated immunity.
- **Hormone regulation:** Hormones, produced by endocrine glands, regulate various biological processes such as growth, metabolism, reproduction, and mood.
- **Apoptosis:** Apoptosis is a programmed cell death process that eliminates damaged or unnecessary cells to maintain tissue homeostasis and remove potential risks.

- **DNA repair:** Cells have mechanisms to repair damaged DNA to maintain the integrity of genetic information and prevent the accumulation of mutations.
- **Blood clotting:** Hemostasis helps prevent excessive bleeding by forming blood clots to seal injured blood vessels.
- **Bone remodeling:** Throughout life, bone tissue undergoes a continuous process of resorption and formation, known as bone remodeling, maintaining bone strength and structure.
- **Cell respiration:** Cells generate energy through cellular respiration, which involves glucose breakdown and ATP production.

These biological processes contribute to the overall function of the human body. It's important to note that this is not an exhaustive list, as the human body is a complex system with numerous interconnected processes occurring simultaneously.

If we dig a little further, we find that physiology is also impacted by exercise and nutrition.

Physiology

If unfamiliar, physiology is a sub-discipline of biology. Biology has a broad focus on the processes and functions of living organisms, while physiology concentrates on HOW the body functions both physically and chemically. Both exercise and nutrition play significant roles in improving physiological function and supporting optimal bodily processes.

When you engage in regular exercise, you challenge your body to work harder and adapt to new demands. This results in various physiological improvements that positively impact your overall function. For example, exercise can increase lung capacity, allowing you to take in more oxygen and improve respiratory efficiency. This, in turn, enhances your endurance and cardiovascular health, making physical tasks feel easier and less taxing on the body.

Exercise promotes improved circulation throughout the body. As you engage in physical activity, your heart pumps more efficiently, delivering oxygen and essential nutrients to your muscles and organs. Enhanced blood flow supports the health of your cardiovascular system and the efficient functioning of various bodily systems.

Regular exercise also stimulates metabolic changes in your body. It can lead to improved metabolism, including increased muscle mass and a higher metabolic rate. This can result in more efficient energy expenditure, improved weight management, and better nutrient utilization. These metabolic improvements contribute to increased energy levels and a greater ability to handle physical demands in your daily life.

In conjunction with exercise, nutrition plays a crucial role in supporting physiological function. Consuming a nutrient-rich diet provides the essential building blocks and fuel for optimal bodily processes. Adequate intake of essential macronutrients (proteins and fats) and micronutrients (vitamins and minerals) supports cellular function, tissue repair, and energy production.

For example, fat is an essential nutrient that provides energy, aids nutrient absorption, supports hormone production, and contributes to cell structure and function. Consuming the right types and amounts of fat is essential for overall health and well-being.

Protein is an essential nutrient that serves as a crucial building block for tissues, organs, enzymes, and hormones in the body. It is necessary for muscle growth and repair, supports a healthy immune system, helps regulate metabolism and hormone production, and plays a role in maintaining overall health and well-being.

Essential vitamins and minerals play vital roles in various physiological functions, such as bone health, immune function, and the synthesis of enzymes and hormones.

The combination of regular exercise and proper nutrition synergistically enhances physiological function. Activity challenges your body to adapt and improve, while food provides the necessary nutrients to support these physiological changes. By incorporating exercise and nutrition into your daily routine, you can optimize physiological function, experience increased energy levels, and better cope with the physical demands of everyday life.

The human body consists of numerous physiological processes that occur to maintain its normal function. Here are some examples of major physiological processes in the human body:

- **Circulation:** The circulatory system, comprised of the heart, blood vessels, and blood, transports oxygen, nutrients, hormones, and other essential substances throughout the body.
- **Respiration:** The respiratory system facilitates the exchange of oxygen and carbon dioxide between the body and the environment. It involves breathing, ventilation of the lungs, and gas exchange in the alveoli.
- **Digestion:** The digestive system breaks down food into smaller molecules, absorbs nutrients, and eliminates waste products. It involves processes such as chewing, swallowing, digestion in the stomach and intestines, and absorption in the small intestine.
- **Excretion:** The excretory system eliminates waste products and toxins from the body. It involves the filtration of blood by the kidneys, resulting in urine formation, which is excreted through the urinary system.
- **Muscular contraction:** Muscles contract and relax to facilitate movement, maintain posture, generate heat, and support various physiological processes.
- **Reproduction:** Reproductive processes involve the production of gametes (sperm and eggs), fertilization, pregnancy, and childbirth, enabling the perpetuation of the species.

It's important to note that this list is not exhaustive, as many more physiological processes occur in the human body. The human body is a complex and interconnected system, with various processes working together to ensure proper functioning.

Then we have neurology.

Neurology

Neurology refers to the processes and functions of the nervous system, which controls the communication and coordination between different parts of your body. Did you guess it also is part of our metabolism?

Neurology plays a crucial role in overall well-being and quality of life. When you engage in regular exercise, you stimulate the release of neurotransmitters in your brain. Neurotransmitters are chemicals that help regulate mood and emotions, such as serotonin and dopamine. Releasing these neurotransmitters during exercise can improve mood, reduce stress, and promote a greater sense of well-being.

Exercise has also been shown to have a positive impact on cognitive function. It can enhance the ability to focus, concentrate, and retain information. Regular physical activity has been associated with improved memory and learning capabilities. This connection is thought to be due to increased blood flow to the brain, which promotes the delivery of oxygen and nutrients essential for optimal brain function. Additionally, exercise stimulates the production of growth factors, such as brain-derived neurotrophic factor (BDNF), which promotes the growth and development of new neurons and strengthens neural connections.

In addition to exercise, nutrition plays a crucial role in supporting neurological function. The brain relies on a steady supply of nutrients to function optimally. Nutrients such as omega-3 fatty acids, B vitamins, antioxidants, and minerals are essential for synthesizing and regulating neurotransmitters, producing energy, and protecting brain cells against oxidative stress and inflammation.

Omega-3 fatty acids, found in fatty fish and other meats, have been associated with improved cognitive function, memory, and mood regulation. Minerals like magnesium and zinc are involved in neuronal signaling and have been linked to improved cognitive function.

A balanced and nutrient-rich diet, along with regular exercise, can have a synergistic effect on neurological function. Combining exercise-induced neurotransmitter release, increased blood flow, and the delivery of essential nutrients through proper nutrition can support optimal brain health, cognitive function, and overall neurological well-being. The human body consists of numerous neurological processes that occur to maintain its normal function. Here is a list of some major neurological processes in the human body:

- **Nerve impulse transmission:** Neurons transmit electrical signals, known as nerve impulses or action potentials, to communicate information within the nervous system and between the nervous system and other body parts.

- **Sensation:** The nervous system detects and processes sensory information from the environment and internal body conditions, allowing us to perceive sensations such as touch, taste, smell, vision, and hearing.

- **Perception:** The brain interprets sensory information from the sensory organs, enabling us to recognize and make sense of the world around us.

- **Motor control:** The nervous system coordinates and controls voluntary and involuntary movements by sending signals from the brain and spinal cord to muscles and glands, allowing us to perform actions and respond to stimuli.

- **Reflexes:** Reflex actions are rapid and involuntary responses to specific stimuli. They are controlled by neural circuits within the spinal cord and are designed to protect the body from harm.

- **Learning and memory:** The nervous system plays a crucial role in learning, memory formation, and retrieval. It involves the strengthening and modification of connections between neurons, known as synaptic plasticity.

- **Emotion and mood regulation:** The nervous system regulates emotions and moods by integrating and processing emotional stimuli, involving brain regions such as the amygdala and prefrontal cortex.

- **Sleep and wakefulness regulation:** The brain controls the sleep-wake cycle, which involves alternating between periods of wakefulness and sleep, including different stages of sleep (e.g., REM sleep and non-REM sleep).

- **Cognitive processes:** The nervous system supports various cognitive functions, including attention, problem-solving, decision-making, language processing, reasoning, and executive functions like planning and inhibition.
- **Neuroplasticity:** The nervous system can reorganize and adapt its structure and function in response to experience, learning, and environmental changes.
- **Neurotransmission:** Neurotransmitters are chemicals released by neurons to transmit signals across synapses, facilitating communication between neurons and disseminating information throughout the nervous system.
- **Neuroendocrine regulation:** The nervous system interacts with the endocrine system to regulate hormone secretion and maintain homeostasis.
- **Pain processing:** The nervous system detects and processes pain signals, enabling us to perceive and respond to painful stimuli.
- **Autonomic nervous system control:** The autonomic nervous system regulates involuntary bodily functions, including heart rate, digestion, respiration, and glandular secretion.
- **Neurodegeneration and neuroprotection:** The nervous system is susceptible to degenerative diseases such as Alzheimer's, Parkinson's, and multiple sclerosis. Neuroprotection refers to mechanisms and processes aimed at preserving the health and function of neurons.

It's important to note that this list is not exhaustive, as many more neurological processes occur in the human body. The human body is a complex and interconnected system, with various processes working together to ensure proper functioning. *This synergy of these combined functions is what makes your metabolism.*

Together, these three systems (your metabolism) are interconnected and work harmoniously to help you achieve optimal health and fitness. By improving your biology, physiology, and neurology (your metabolism) through regular exercise and proper nutrition, you can improve your quality of life and reduce the risk of chronic disease.

I emphasize that this is a unique journey for you and becoming the best version of YOU. I must remind you that this is not a group project. My story is full of examples of how it all came down to me. No excuses, no crutches. So, before we explore the F2 Method, it is crucial to set the stage and examine the importance of individuality, both biological and psychological.

Bio-Individuality

I want to get this one out first. **Just because you're different doesn't mean you're different.**

It's popular for people to invoke bio individuality when claiming why one particular protocol, product, supplement, or bio-hack is *better* for some people than others. The idea that you have a different biological makeup and need different things based on your genetics, some irregular hormone deficiency, an inability to process a specific amino acid, et cetera, is utter nonsense.

There, I said it. Nonsense.

Bio-individuality has become a marketing term used by companies and influencers to establish a need based on fictional, scientific mumbo jumbo that makes people think they are at risk if they don't buy into the hype…or their product.

What bio-individuality actually means is that the **individual's total experience determines the intervention's effective scope.**

We're all born with the same biological needs. Your biology is that of a human being. The basics of human function and survival are consistent across the board. The biological systems you were born with are the same as almost every other human being on the planet. To name a few:

- Oxygenated blood is red.
- Hair grows from roots.
- Carbohydrates are non-essential nutrients.
- Muscles need protein to grow.

- Hormones control metabolism.
- Sleep is a requirement for health.

And on and on.

Bio-individuality is the result of your life's exposure and experiences. This includes how you lived growing up, the things you did, the food you ate, your family life, and the emotions or stresses you lived through. Everything has an impact on your metabolic function. That means not just your biology but your physiology and neurology too.

Bio-individuality encompasses your lifestyle habits, preferences, and ability to process change. The way you live your life impacts your health. The interventions you need to apply to improve your health may require changes that affect your routine more than your actual biology.

Bio-individuality includes your mindset, belief systems, and world views. Often the challenges you face are not physical or biological. Many of the solutions you will find in life come from changing how you think about and view situations and developing an awareness of your limitations and potential.

Bio-individuality is not an excuse for why something isn't working for you. Something isn't working for you because you haven't established the basis of core function and health in the three Quality of Life Domains. The solution to improving health must start at the core level of human need **before** it enters the realm of bio-individuality.

This is the single biggest mistake people make on their journey. The root cause of stalls, wasted time, frustration, and eventual failure is not ensuring that the basics of human needs are met consistently before expanding the process of improving health to other areas. Too frequently, the additional stress, complexity, cost, or time commitment required to maintain that depth of focus is unsustainable.

Do not use bio-individuality as a crutch to hold onto unhealthy habits. Do not use bio-individuality as an excuse for why you're failing. Own your journey. Acknowledge your core human needs first and see what happens when you take care of those.

Now let's talk about biomechanical individuality.

Biomechanical Individuality

Biomechanical individuality refers to the fact that each individual has unique physical characteristics that affect their ability to perform exercises and activities. These physical characteristics include body type, limb length, joint structure, and muscle fiber composition. These characteristics can impact your biomechanics or how your body moves and functions during physical activity.

Biomechanical individuality means that not every exercise or training program will work for every person. For example, an individual with longer limbs may have a different range of motion and muscle activation during a squat compared to an individual with shorter limbs. Similarly, an individual with a different muscle fiber composition may respond differently to strength training compared to another individual.

If we take the example of doing squats, biomechanical individuality can impact squat technique in several ways. For example:

- **Body type:** Someone with a longer torso may have a different squat technique compared to those with a shorter torso. Those with a longer torso may tend to lean forward more during the squat, while those with a shorter torso may be able to maintain a more upright posture.
- **Limb length:** Someone with longer legs may have a different range of motion during the squat compared to those with shorter legs. For example, those with longer legs may need to widen their stance to achieve proper depth, while those with shorter legs may be able to keep a narrower stance.
- **Joint structure:** Hip or knee joint structure differences can impact squat technique. For example, someone with greater hip external rotation may be able to maintain a more open-foot position during the squat. In contrast, those with limited hip mobility may need a more closed-foot position.

Understanding biomechanical individuality is essential in designing effective and safe training programs. Fitness professionals must consider your unique physical characteristics when prescribing exercises and programming to ensure that exercises are safe and effective for the individual. This may involve modifying exercises to account for differences in limb length or joint structure or adjusting training volume and intensity for differences in muscle fiber composition and recovery ability.

Understanding the factors of biomechanical individuality is vital in determining the optimal exercise program and proper techniques for individuals. Further, when you understand your biomechanical uniqueness, you will know why certain exercises work better for you than others and can avoid unnecessary frustrations.

Your individual health and fitness goals will be restricted or boosted based on your metabolism. Your metabolism can change and be different from those around you. The conversation about metabolism is so important that it needs its own chapter. So, let's dive in!

Individual Variation in Body Composition

The journey of changing one's body composition, which involves gaining lean mass and losing body fat, is deeply personal and varied among individuals. This variability is influenced by several factors:

- **Genetic Predisposition**: Genetics play a significant role in determining how easily one can gain muscle or lose fat. Some individuals may find it easier to develop lean muscle mass due to their genetic makeup, while others may struggle more with weight loss or muscle gain.
- **Hormonal Influences**: Hormones significantly influence body composition. Testosterone, for example, aids in muscle building. Variations in hormonal levels can greatly affect one's ability to gain lean mass or lose fat.
- **Metabolic Rate:** Everyone has a unique metabolism, which is the performance of how your body functions. A better-performing

metabolism can facilitate fat loss, while an inefficient one might make it more challenging.

- **Age and Sex**: As we age, changes in muscle mass and fat distribution occur. Additionally, men and women tend to accumulate fat differently and also differ in muscle development due to hormonal differences.
- **Lifestyle Factors**: Diet, exercise, stress levels, and sleep quality significantly influence body composition. Nutritional choices and physical activity levels can accelerate or impede progress in altering body composition.
- **Health Conditions**: Certain medical conditions and medications can impact weight and muscle mass. Conditions like hypothyroidism or insulin resistance can make weight management more challenging.

Gaining Lean Mass

Gaining lean muscle mass requires a combination of strength training and appropriate nutrition. However, the response to training and diet varies. Some individuals may see rapid muscle growth with specific exercise regimens, while others may require more time and varied approaches to see similar results. Nutritional needs, particularly protein intake, also differ based on individual body types and activity levels.

Beyond the Caloric Equation

While a fuel macronutrient deficit is essential for fat loss, the process is more complex than just calories in versus calories out. Factors like the type of food consumed, the timing of meals, and individual metabolic responses play crucial roles. Furthermore, how the body responds to different forms of exercise—such as cardiovascular activities versus resistance training—can vary significantly from person to person.

Consistency and Adaptation

Regardless of the starting point, consistency in diet and exercise is key to changing body composition. However, it's also important to adapt strategies over time. What works initially might not be as effective as the body adapts. Regularly evaluating and modifying exercise routines and dietary habits can help overcome plateaus and continue progress.

Embracing Individuality in Body Transformation

Understanding and embracing individual differences is crucial in the journey of altering body composition. It's important to avoid comparing one's progress with others and to focus on personal improvements and health. By recognizing and adapting to these individual variations, one can effectively work towards their specific goals of gaining lean mass and losing body fat, keeping in mind that the journey is as unique as the individual themselves.

The Impact of Medications

When discussing the complexities of altering body composition, gaining lean mass, and losing body fat, it's crucial to consider the role of medications. Pharmaceuticals can significantly influence these processes, often in ways that are not immediately apparent.

Medications and Metabolic Rate

- **Impact on Metabolism:** Certain medications can affect the body's metabolic performance. For example, some thyroid medications increase energy expenditure, potentially aiding in weight loss, while others can stimulate fuel storage, making weight gain more likely.

- **Appetite and Food Intake:** Some drugs can alter appetite, either suppressing or stimulating it. This change in appetite can lead to increased or decreased food intake, subsequently affecting body composition.

Hormonal Alterations and Body Composition

- **Hormonal Therapies:** Medications like hormonal replacement therapy or birth control can alter the body's hormonal balance, impacting the ability to gain muscle or lose fat. These hormonal changes can also affect where the body stores fat.
- **Insulin Sensitivity:** Medications that affect insulin sensitivity, such as those for diabetes, can have a direct impact on how the body processes sugars and stores fat.

Medication-Induced Fluid Retention

Some medications cause the body to retain fluid, which can affect body weight and composition. This retention might not be actual fat gain but can impact measurements and how the body looks and feels.

Effects on Muscle Mass

- **Muscle Growth and Repair:** Certain medications can interfere with muscle growth and repair. For example, long-term use of corticosteroids can lead to muscle wasting.
- **Exercise Response:** Some drugs may affect how the body responds to exercise, either enhancing or diminishing the effectiveness of physical activity in building muscle or burning fat.
- **Exercise Tolerance:** Medications can influence energy levels and exercise tolerance, affecting one's ability to engage in physical activity.

- **Nutrient Absorption:** Certain drugs can impact the absorption of nutrients essential for muscle growth and fat loss, like protein, vitamins, and minerals.

Navigating Medication Effects with Healthcare Providers

It's important to have open discussions with healthcare providers about the potential impacts of medications on body composition goals. Adjustments to medication regimes or additional strategies might be necessary to mitigate unwanted effects.

Incorporating the impact of medications into the discussion of body composition underscores the complexity of this journey. It's not just about diet and exercise; it's also about understanding and managing the broader influences on your body, including the effects of medications. By considering these factors and working closely with healthcare professionals, individuals can create a more effective and holistic plan to achieve their body composition goals.

Your Individual Context

Determining your individual context is pivotal for making informed choices that improve your quality of life. This process involves acknowledging the intricate interplay of genetic predispositions, hormonal influences, and metabolic rates, which significantly dictate how one gains lean mass or loses body fat. It also requires considering the impact of lifestyle factors like diet and exercise, and understanding the profound influence of medications on your body's response to these changes. Recognizing biomechanical individuality highlights the importance of tailoring exercise and nutrition plans to your unique physical characteristics.

By comprehensively evaluating these diverse elements, you can develop a personalized approach that aligns with your body's specific needs and goals. This holistic understanding not only steers you towards more effective strategies for altering body composition but also lays a strong foundation for enhancing your overall well-being, ensuring that the path to improved quality of life is as unique and individualized as you are.

Now that you have a foundational understanding of how your individuality plays a crucial role in optimal health, we can get into the nuts and bolts of what the F2 Method is. The F2 Method gives you a framework to use for the rest of your life. If you pay attention, you will learn how to avoid stalls and plateaus, and live the most independent and body confident life you can imagine.

Takeaways

- Health, fitness, an sickness are measure of the same things
- Your metabolism is the complete function of your entire body, not just how you burn energy
- Individuality isn't found in your genetics as much as it is in your background, lifestyle, and environment.
- How you look as you change your body composition is unique to you. That doesn't impact your ability to change your body composition.
- You have to understand what you want to change and why. Without this information, nothing you try will work for very long.

Resources

- Get **FREE** Bonus material that includes a complete breakdown and analysis of the most common fitness and nutrition programs to help you evaluate which ones will work best for you by following the F2 Method.
- Join **Coach Bronson's Body Confident Support Group** on Discord and meet more people who are improving themselves every day. https://discord.coachbronson.com
- Download the **FREE Body Confident Book Bonus Material** and Community information at https://bodyconfidentbook.com.

CHAPTER 3

THE F2 METHOD

*"The F2 Method is a **holistic** evaluation of an **individual's** lifestyle, environment, and goals, using an understanding of evidence-based health **concepts and principles** to build a **sustainable** plan that **measurably** improves your quality of life."*
~ Coach Bronson

The F2 Method is a framework that guides the evaluation process of successful lifestyle planning. This framework ensures that you create a personalized plan tailored to your individual needs and goals while increasing the chance of long-term sustainability and success.

The F2 Method is built on the idea that how you think about a problem will guide how you solve that problem. Its goal is to remove bias and support the honest collection of data that leads to applicable and appropriate solutions. If the F2 Method is followed, when you use it, you will end up with a specific solution to help you reach your individual goals.

The F2 Method is broken down into five core concepts that help guide the Quality of Life Domains of mindset, fitness, and nutrition. For each domain, there are three tenets to follow for optimal health. The methodology starts with these overarching core concepts.

Five Core Concepts

Five concepts make the F2 Method work. They are the paradigms that form the thought process and foundation for filtering through the abundance of health information available into sustainable actions. They are:

- Prioritize individual goals.
- Get the whole picture.
- Follow concepts, not rules.
- Make solutions sustainable.
- Measure and evaluate.

As you read more about each core concept, remember they are your home base. No matter what happens along the way, if you return to these five things, you can reset, re-evaluate, and start moving forward.

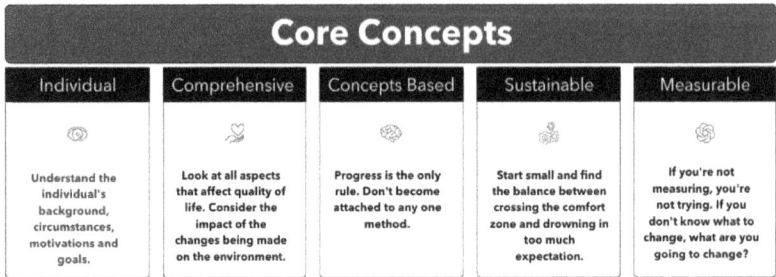

Core Concepts

Individual	Comprehensive	Concepts Based	Sustainable	Measurable
Understand the individual's background, circumstances, motivations and goals.	Look at all aspects that affect quality of life. Consider the impact of the changes being made on the environment.	Progress is the only rule. Don't become attached to any one method.	Start small and find the balance between crossing the comfort zone and drowning in too much expectation.	If you're not measuring, you're not trying. If you don't know what to change, what are you going to change?

Image 3 – Core Concepts

The core concepts are your foundation. From there, you build the legs of the stool with your mindset, fitness, and nutrition—your Quality of Life Domains.

Quality of Life Domains

The F2 Method is a strategy for making sense of information to inform decision-making. It sets the groundwork for thought processes involved in creating plans of action. However, to fully utilize it, you need to understand the who, what, where, and why of the remaining components. Specifically, where do you apply these actions? Which aspects of life should you focus on for change? And why is it important?

Understanding the five elements of the F2 Method is a good beginning. Still, without comprehending how the quality of life is constructed, you might be unsure which parts should be in place and how to link them correctly.

> *"Quality of life, the degree to which an individual is healthy, comfortable, and able to participate in or enjoy life events... Within the arena of health care, quality of life is viewed as multidimensional, encompassing emotional, physical, material, and social well-being."* ~ Jenkinson, Quality of Life

Interpreting this, we can say that quality of life includes your health, physical capacity, mental well-being, and ability to socialize and participate in various activities. In essence, people often associate quality of life with mental, physical, and biological factors influencing day-to-day living. While you may not discuss your biology frequently, you talk about your health. Mental health is primarily governed by overall health. Health as a broad concept is intricately connected with fitness, another critical component shaping the quality of life.

To understand and improve quality of life, we can translate these broad concepts into three practical domains or areas of focus. These domains form the foundation for enhancing your quality of life. They are:

- **Mindset Domain:** This domain includes self-awareness, future vision, identity, perception of self and the world, belief systems, and habits.
- **Fitness Domain:** This domain refers to your body's performance. It covers your body's capacity to work, recover, and handle external stress.
- **Nutrition Domain:** This domain involves your body's functionality. It represents how efficiently your body operates, supporting physical performance by managing internal stress.

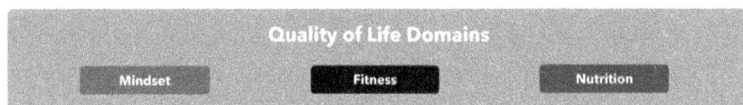

Image 4 - Quality of Life Domains

Mindset focuses on your thought processes, while fitness and nutrition focus on your Systems of Function or metabolism. By focusing on these three domains, you can effectively deconstruct the idea of quality of life into smaller tangible pieces. You now have the link between health concepts and how your lifestyle affects your quality of life.

For each domain, you are guided by three tenets. There are nine total tenets.

The Nine Tenets of Health

Each of these categories contains a set of foundational concepts to keep you moving in the right direction. Let's call them Tenets of Health. If you are missing any one of these, your progress will falter, and things will be more challenging for you than they need to be.

Many focus heavily on one or two tenets in the Systems of Function (fitness and nutrition) and rarely address anything in thought processes (mindset). This is why you get stuck, frustrated, and have difficulty being consistent. You need all Nine Tenets of Health to fully realize your best life.

- **Tenets One Through Three** - Your mindset is guided by:
    - o Know your WHY
    - o Know You
    - o Know How
- **Tenets Four Through Six** - Fitness is guided by:
    - o Move Well
    - o Move Weight
    - o Move Often
- **Tenets Seven Through Nine** - Nutrition is guided by:
    - o Nutrient Density

o   Bioavailability
o   Satiety

The diagram shows you what the F2 Method looks like when each component is incorporated into the whole. Each element contributes to your lifestyle choices, which ultimately affects the individual (you).

Now that you have a foundation in the methodology, let's delve into each component for a better understanding. We will begin with the five core concepts.

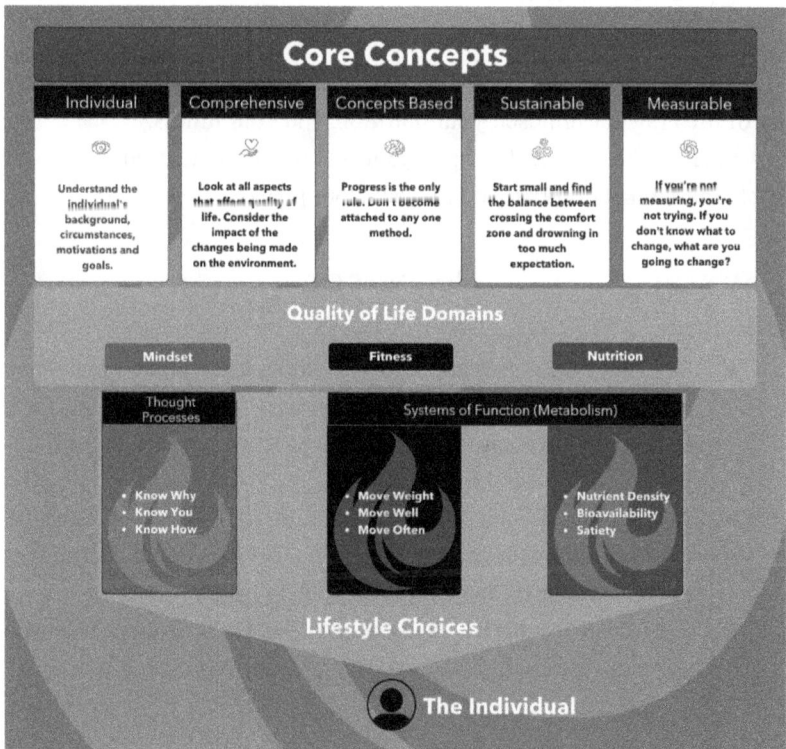

Core Concepts

Individual	Comprehensive	Concepts Based	Sustainable	Measurable
Understand the individual's background, circumstances, motivations and goals.	Look at all aspects that affect quality of life. Consider the impact of the changes being made on the environment.	Progress is the only rule. Don't become attached to any one method.	Start small and find the balance between crossing the comfort zone and drowning in too much expectation.	If you're not measuring, you're not trying. If you don't know what to change, what are you going to change?

Quality of Life Domains

Mindset	Fitness	Nutrition
Thought Processes	Systems of Function (Metabolism)	
• Know Why • Know You • Know How	• Move Weight • Move Well • Move Often	• Nutrient Density • Bioavailability • Satiety

Lifestyle Choices

The Individual

Takeaways

Remember, nothing you do will work as well or last as long if you don't meet these five criteria for success.

- Prioritize individual goals.
- Get the whole picture.
- Follow concepts, not rules.
- Make solutions sustainable.
- Measure and evaluate.

The three main areas that you need to focus on to build a better quality of life are your mindset, your nutrition, and your fitness.

Each of those areas has specific tenets to follow that will help you apply the right actions for you to reach your goals.

Resources

- Get **FREE** Bonus material that includes a complete breakdown and analysis of the most common fitness and nutrition programs to help you evaluate which ones will work best for you by following the F2 Method.
- Join **Coach Bronson's Body Confident Support Group** on Discord and meet more people who are improving themselves every day. https://discord.coachbronson.com
- Download the **FREE Body Confident Book Bonus Material** and Community information at https://bodyconfidentbook.com.

CHAPTER 4

~~~~~~

THE FIVE CORE CONCEPTS

*"If you change the way you look at things, the
things you look at change." ~ Wayne Dyer*

The five core concepts are your foundation. Whenever in doubt about your health and well-being, fall back to your five core concepts. You will start with self-reflection and finding that starting point to set individualized goals.

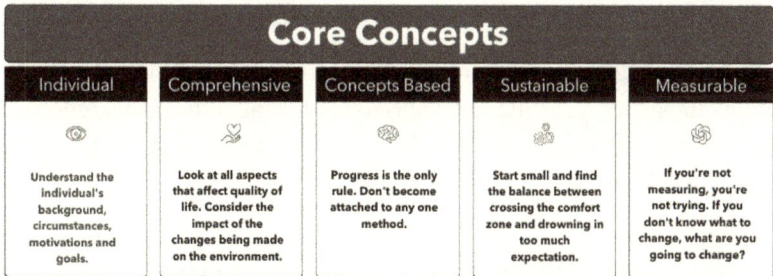

Core Concepts

Individual	Comprehensive	Concepts Based	Sustainable	Measurable
Understand the individual's background, circumstances, motivations and goals.	Look at all aspects that affect quality of life. Consider the impact of the changes being made on the environment.	Progress is the only rule. Don't become attached to any one method.	Start small and find the balance between crossing the comfort zone and drowning in too much expectation.	If you're not measuring, you're not trying. If you don't know what to change, what are you going to change?

Image 3 – Core Concepts

Concept One: Prioritize Individual Goals

The F2 Method is built on a belief that individual goals must be the priority. Everyone is unique, and there is no one-size-fits-all solution for health and fitness.

Nothing can happen without understanding where you want to go; when you want to get there; and what you can do to make it happen. This information is crucial in developing a personalized plan that will lead to success.

Success requires a Why, a Goal, and a Timeline. These set the tone for every decision and adjustment along the way. Each of these is different for everyone and will change over time. Self-awareness and constant evaluation of your journey are integral to sustained success.

Ask yourself:

- Do you have a *Why*?
- What aspects of your lifestyle are contributing to your health or sickness?
- What limiting beliefs do you have about health or fitness?
- What are you ready, willing, and able to do?
- Do you have something you're not willing to give up?
- What is the lifestyle you want to live?
- What are the things you need to do to maintain that lifestyle?
- Do you have physical limitations to remove from your life?

Answering these questions and more will give you a clear view of the things impacting your life and your vision for the future. This reflection sets the foundation for how you interpret the information out there and apply your individual context to your courses of action.

Concept Two: Get the Whole Picture

There is a lot of information in this book because there are a lot of things that can impact your progress. Not only are there physical, biological, and mental things affecting your life, but emotions, environment, and relationships play a role too.

Any solution to help you move forward has to include tools to address as many of these factors as possible. It will be harder to do if you don't consider your sleep when trying to build muscle. If you don't account for stress from work, you'll be frustrated when you feel worn down, and it's harder to work out at the end of the week. Anxiety about spending the weekend with your in-laws might trigger cravings. How do you handle that?

No solution is linear. Every problem is different. Most issues have layers and layers to them. Often, addressing the first thing isn't what moves you forward. The more questions you ask, the more answers you get and the better picture you have of what's truly going on.

Consider the following:

- Health history
- Diet history
- Physical limitations
- Medications
- Stressors (physical, mental, biological, environmental)
- Habit loops and triggers
- Relationships
- Finances
- Schedule and Responsibilities

Ask questions and understand the scope of things that play a role in your behavior and mental and physical states so you can better identify changes that can significantly impact your progress.

Concept Three:
Follow Concepts, Not Rules

The F2 Method is not about following a specific program or guideline. Instead, it is based on the concepts of health, fitness, nutrition, and mindset that have provided the greatest flexibility and results in all clients I've worked with over the last ten years.

Why something is working is more important than the thing itself. A common misconception is that the *thing*—a nutrition plan, an exercise plan, or a product—is the magic behind your success. It's not the thing; it's what you did that was different. For example, you go on a whole-food Keto diet and lose a ton of weight. You think Keto was the secret.

It wasn't. Keto is the thing that helps you to remove processed food, increase protein intake, get more nutrients, and eat less.

If you had gone Paleo or Carnivore, you would have had the same results.

Your actions to change how your body functions are more important than the box you put them into. There are a million programs out there that work. Most of them work for many of the same reasons. The concepts of how the human body functions are universal to all humans, **regardless of what name we give them**.

Avoid developing an emotional connection to, or basing your identity on, any hard and fast guidelines or rules. The more you eliminate options outside what's working right now, the more you limit yourself when those things stop working—**and they will stop working.**

You are not *Low-Carb*, *Keto*, or *Carnivore*; you are following a diet that identifies as such.

Whether you do CrossFit, follow a High-Intensity Training (HIT) program, or Powerlifting doesn't matter. Are you moving closer to your goals? That's all that matters.

Your progress is the only rule.

There are many different ideas and methods of approaching aspects of health and fitness. That's the way it should be. Each person will need at least a dozen variations at some point. Who wants to stick with one?

When you follow concepts instead of rules, you realize that the habit is more important than the action. Being consistent in doing things to improve your health will always move you forward, even if it's not the 100% *best* way of doing it.

When you focus on how your progress is affected first, you stop looking for *the best way*. Instead, you start looking for the way that works for you. In time, you realize there are no absolutes, only what's effective for now.

Concept Four:
Make Solutions Sustainable

A great way to describe accessibility is by grabbing the *low-hanging fruit*—the easiest to grab.

What gets you doing more than you've done, but isn't so far outside your comfort zone that you're fighting yourself every day to do it? Finding this level of progress is what I call the 1% Rule. I know I said not to follow any rules—it's my book! This one is okay to follow.

Obviously, it's not a literal one percent, but the takeaway is that it only takes a little bit more. To do something you've never done, you have to do something you've never done. That is how it works.

Any action plan should help improve the situation, not make it worse. Don't do too many things at once; don't do something so big that the disruption to your life and those around you is counterproductive.

Just start:

- Walking more
- Parking further away
- Taking the stairs
- Picking up something heavy a few times a day
- Practicing getting down and up off the floor

Progress comes from going outside your comfort zone. Anywhere over that line will move the needle. Avoid big leaps. Take small steps. You'll make more progress, it will stick better, and it will last longer.

Concept Five: Measure and Evaluate

The only way to know if you're making progress is to measure and evaluate regularly. That's why I emphasize the importance of tracking progress and evaluating results regularly.

Making changes and adjustments without accurate and meaningful data is impossible. If you are considering all aspects of your quality of life, there is no limit to the number of things you can measure to gauge your progress.

The idea of tracking can be overwhelming. There is so much data, and tracking everything can seem complicated and time-consuming. Like everything else in the F2 Method, sustainable habits should be emphasized. If you're following the previous four areas discussed in the method, you know there is no requirement for how, what, or when you measure as long as whatever you do is working.

The main point is the more you keep an eye on what you're doing and how it affects you, the more chances you have at success. There are two things to measure. First is anything that affects your biology, neurology, or physiology that can be measured. Second is what those effects actually are.

For example, look at lifting weights. The weight being lifted is a thing (stimulus or stressor) you can measure. The speed you can move the weight, muscle size, and the ability to move a heavier weight are measures of weightlifting's change on your body.

There are many ways to keep track of how things are going. If you're following the method correctly, there should never be an issue or concern with stalling or plateauing. With all the aspects of health and well-being involved in reaching your goals, even if one thing stops progressing, ten more will keep moving forward.

Tracking allows you to make adjustments more accurately, proves that you're moving in the right direction, and assures you that things are going as planned.

Now, you may wonder, *if this is a method, where are the steps?*

The number of variations in how to develop a lifestyle solution to meet each person where they are is far too many to put into a book. That's why the F2 Method is based on concepts, not rules.

If you integrate the five core concepts of the F2 Method into your process, you will stay on a path that moves you in the right direction at a reasonable, safe, and sustainable level. The paradigm the method creates gives you a set of parameters that prevent enormous miscalculations or errors in judgment.

We will explore affecting change a bit later. For now, let's explore the Quality of Life Domains in detail.

Takeaways

The five core concepts of the F2 Method are summed up in this one statement.

- *"The F2 Method is a holistic evaluation of an individual's lifestyle, environment, and goals, using an understanding of evidence-based health concepts and principles to build a sustainable plan that measurably improves your quality of life."*

Resources

- Get **FREE** Bonus material that includes a complete breakdown and analysis of the most common fitness and nutrition programs to help you evaluate which ones will work best for you by following the F2 Method.
- Join **Coach Bronson's Body Confident Support Group** on Discord and meet more people who are improving themselves every day. https://discord.coachbronson.com
- Download the **FREE Body Confident Book Bonus Material** and Community information at https://bodyconfidentbook.com.

CHAPTER 5

- -

QUALITY OF LIFE DOMAINS: THE OPTIMAL HEALTH TRIFECTA

"A healthy outside starts from the inside."
~ Robert Urich

Only recently have we seen a push to incorporate a holistic approach to health. Historically, we work to address a symptom. High cholesterol? Change your diet, exercise—or do both and take a pill. Overweight? Same remedy. What we have failed to do is look at the root cause of these symptoms. If you look at the three domains, each provides a window into the actions you take in your everyday life that affect your health, fitness, and quality of life. These domains contain areas of thought that direct your efforts, develop habits, and increase your potential for success. Your lifestyle, decisions, and actions link each domain to an aspect of your quality of life.

How you live your life determines how well the life is that you live.

In other words, it's about your lifestyle. Lifestyle can be broken into two categories: thought processes and systems of function. Your thoughts and actions impact your body, mind, environment, relationships, and other factors affecting your life.

> *"Quality of life, the degree to which an individual is healthy, comfortable, and able to participate in or enjoy life events . . . Within the arena of health care,*

quality of life is viewed as multidimensional, encom-
passing emotional, physical, material, and social
well-being."~ Jenkinson, Quality of Life

Interpreting this, we can say that quality of life includes your health, physical capacity, mental well-being, and ability to socialize and participate in various activities. In essence, people often associate quality of life with mental, physical, and biological factors that influence day-to-day living.

The Quality of Life Domains give you a playbook you can apply to your life. They are high-level concepts you can use to determine if your lifestyle is doing you more harm than good. It all starts with your mindset.

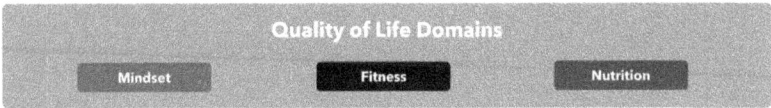

Quality of Life Domains

| Mindset | Fitness | Nutrition |

- **The Mindset Domain:** The most important domain is Mindset. This domain relates to your **thought processes**. It includes self-awareness, future vision, identity, perception of self and the world, belief systems, and habits. Your mental and emotional well-being significantly impacts your ability to maintain a healthy lifestyle. Even the most well-designed fitness and nutrition plans can falter without the right mindset. *Your mind controls everything.*

   Cultivating a positive mindset that encourages consistency, resilience, and self-compassion is essential. This might involve addressing limiting beliefs, setting achievable goals, or developing healthy habits supporting your journey to optimal health. By focusing on mindset, you build a strong foundation for lasting change.

- **The Fitness Domain:** Fitness encompasses how well the body can function in various aspects, including strength, endurance, flexibility, and balance. This domain refers to your body's performance. It covers your body's capacity to work, recover, and handle external stress. Each individual's fitness goals and needs may vary, which is why it's essential to assess your current fitness level, goals, and personal preferences to create a customized workout plan that works for you. For example, you may want to build muscle mass versus improving your cardiovascular performance. There are differences in how to train for each goal. By considering the unique fitness requirements and objectives, you can develop a targeted plan that addresses specific needs, making it more likely that you'll stick to it and see results.

- **The Nutrition Domain:** Nutrition plays a vital role in supporting the body's functions and overall well-being. This domain involves your body's functionality. It represents how efficiently your body operates, supporting physical performance by managing internal stress. It's important to remember that no single diet works for everyone. Just as with fitness, each individual has different nutritional needs and preferences. Understanding your unique dietary requirements and the most effective nutrition for your body's optimal health is essential. This might involve making simple changes to your existing diet, incorporating more nutrient-dense foods, or even developing an entirely new meal plan. By focusing on your specific nutritional needs, you create a sustainable and enjoyable way of eating that supports your health and fitness goals.

Understanding The Mindset Domain

Remember that your thinking habits dictate your life habits. Developing a mindset for success takes practice. Your mindset is crucial for your health journey because it lays the groundwork for your overall well-being and success in reaching your goals. Here's why it matters:

- **Motivation and Commitment:** Your mindset keeps you motivated and committed to your health journey. It gives you the drive and determination to stay focused, even when faced with challenges or setbacks. With a positive mindset, you can stay dedicated to your goals and keep moving forward.

- **Goal Setting and Clarity:** Developing a clear mindset helps you set meaningful goals and establish a vision for your health journey. It allows you to define what you want to achieve, understand why it's important, and figure out how to get there. This clarity helps guide your decisions and actions.

- **Self-Awareness and Personal Growth:** The mindset domain emphasizes self-awareness, which means understanding your thoughts, emotions, strengths, weaknesses, and values. By being self-aware, you can identify any limiting beliefs, self-sabotaging behaviors, or negative thought patterns that might hinder your progress. This awareness opens the door to personal growth and transformation.

- **Resilience and Stress Management:** Cultivating a healthy mindset equips you with resilience and effective stress management skills. It allows you to navigate stressful situations, setbacks, and obstacles that may arise during your health journey. With a positive mindset, you can bounce back, learn from challenges, and maintain an optimistic outlook.

- **Mind-Body Connection:** The mindset domain recognizes the strong connection between your mind and body. A positive mindset promotes mental well-being, reduces stress levels, and can positively impact your physical health. It encourages behaviors that contribute to your overall well-being, such as self-care, managing your emotions, and prioritizing your mental and emotional health.

- **Sustainable Lifestyle Habits:** A healthy mindset encourages you to adopt sustainable lifestyle habits rather than pursuing short-term or unsustainable approaches. It helps you develop a positive relationship with your body, food, exercise, and overall self-care. By fostering a long-term perspective, a healthy mindset supports the creation of lasting habits that can be maintained for a lifetime.

By focusing on your mindset, you can cultivate a positive, empowered, and resilient mental outlook that propels you forward on your health journey. This not only increases your chances of achieving your goals but also contributes to your overall well-being, happiness, and fulfillment.

How to Improve Your Mindset

- Begin by cultivating self-awareness and understanding your current mindset and belief systems.
- Assess your motivations, values, and aspirations to create a future vision for yourself.
- Set specific goals aligned with your vision to help establish a clear direction.
- Develop strategies and habits that support a positive mindset, consistency, resilience, and self-compassion.
- Regular self-reflection and evaluation enable you to monitor your progress and adjust as needed.

When you set your mind right, you can better focus on the fitness and nutrition system functions. The fitness domain directly supports the mindset domain. If unfamiliar, exercise doesn't only impact our physical health. It can affect hormones, which affect mood and mental health.

Understanding Fitness

Your fitness is crucial to your health journey because it directly impacts your physical well-being, strength, endurance, and metabolic function. Here's why it matters to you:

- **Physical Health and Disease Prevention:** Engaging in regular physical activity and exercise through the fitness domain promotes optimal physical health. It helps reduce the risk of chronic diseases such as heart disease, diabetes, and certain cancers. Regular exercise supports a healthy cardiovascular system, strengthens bones and muscles, improves lung function, and enhances overall bodily functions.

- **Strength and Functional Abilities:** Increases a focus on building strength, essential for performing daily activities, maintaining good posture, and preventing injuries. Strength training exercises improve muscle tone, increase bone density, and enhance joint stability. Having a strong body enables you to engage in various physical activities with ease and reduces the risk of age-related declines in functional abilities.
- **Endurance and Energy Levels:** Regular exercise improves cardiovascular fitness and enhances your body's ability to use oxygen efficiently. This increases endurance, stamina, and energy levels, allowing you to engage in physical activities for extended periods without feeling fatigued. Improved endurance also supports better performance in sports, recreational activities, and daily tasks.
- **Mental Well-being and Stress Reduction:** Engaging in physical activity has numerous mental health benefits. Exercise releases endorphins, which are natural mood-enhancing chemicals in the brain, leading to improved mood, reduced stress levels, and increased well-being. Regular exercise can also help alleviate symptoms of anxiety and depression, boost self-confidence, and improve cognitive function.
- **Body Composition and Weight Management:** Fitness plays a significant role in body composition, which refers to the ratio of muscle, fat, and other tissues in your body. Regular exercise, combined with proper nutrition, helps build lean muscle mass, improve body composition, and support healthy weight management. Physical activity increases energy expenditure, helping you maintain a healthy weight or achieve weight loss goals.
- **Longevity and Quality of Life:** Engaging in regular exercise and maintaining fitness levels have been linked to increased longevity and improved quality of life. Regular physical activity can delay the onset of age-related health conditions, improve

mobility and independence, enhance cognitive function, and contribute to an overall higher quality of life as you age.

By incorporating fitness into your health journey, you can reap these benefits and enjoy a stronger, healthier, and more vibrant life. Regular exercise and physical activity not only contribute to your physical well-being but also have a positive impact on your mental, emotional, and overall holistic health.

How to Improve Your Fitness

- Evaluate your current fitness level and identify areas for improvement.
- Learn about proper movement techniques to ensure safety and maximize the effectiveness of exercises.
- Focus on consistency and establish a workout routine that aligns with your goals and preferences.
- Gradually increase intensity levels, challenging your body appropriately to stimulate adaptations without exceeding your capabilities.
- Seek guidance from a trainer or coach to assess your workouts, select appropriate weights, and learn proper intensity levels.
- Monitoring progress, tracking performance, and adjusting the workout plan as needed allows the individual to improve continuously.

Finally, for optimal health, we have to consider nutrition.

Understanding Nutrition

Your nutrition is critically important to your health journey because it directly affects your overall well-being, energy levels, disease prevention, and the functioning of your body. Here's why it matters to you:

- **Nutrient Intake and Optimal Function:** Proper nutrition provides your body with essential nutrients, including macronutrients (carbohydrates, proteins, and fats) and micronutrients (vitamins and minerals). These nutrients are the building blocks for all bodily functions, supporting optimal cellular function, organ health, and overall physiological processes. This ensures your body has the necessary resources to function at its best.

- **Disease Prevention and Immune Function:** A nutrient-rich diet plays a crucial role in preventing chronic diseases, such as heart disease, diabetes, obesity, and certain cancers. Nutrients from whole foods support a robust immune system, helping your body defend against infections and illnesses and promoting faster recovery.

- **Energy Levels and Optimal Performance:** Nutrition directly impacts your energy levels and overall performance. The foods you consume provide the fuel your body needs for daily activities, exercise, and mental tasks. A nutrient-rich diet improves mental clarity and supports physical performance. Proper nutrition also enhances exercise performance, maximizing the benefits of your fitness activities.

- **Body Composition and Weight Management:** Nutrition plays a significant role in body composition and weight management. Proper nutrition and regular physical activity help maintain a healthy weight, promote fat loss, and build lean muscle mass. Consuming the right balance of macronutrients and controlling portion sizes supports healthy body composition goals, reduces the risk of obesity-related health issues, and improves overall body image and self-confidence.

- **Gut Health and Digestion:** The foods you eat influence the health of your digestive system and gut microbiota. This is essential for proper digestion, nutrient absorption, and overall gut health. A healthy gut contributes to improved immune function, reduces the risk of gastrointestinal disorders, and promotes overall well-being.

- **Mental and Emotional Well-being:** Nutrition significantly impacts your mental and emotional well-being. Certain nutrients, such as omega-3 fatty acids, B vitamins, and antioxidants, support brain health, cognitive function, and mood regulation. A diet with these nutrients can help reduce the risk of mental health disorders, improve focus and concentration, and enhance overall emotional well-being.

By prioritizing nutrition in your health journey, you can nourish your body with the essential nutrients it needs to thrive. Making informed food choices and incorporating various nutrient-dense foods contribute to improved overall health, disease prevention, optimal functioning, and a higher quality of life. Remember, nutrition is not just about restriction; it's about nourishing and fueling your body for optimal performance and well-being.

How to Improve Your Nutrition

- Assess your current eating habits and nutritional choices.
- Prioritize nutrient-dense foods, and focus on providing the body with essential vitamins, minerals, and beneficial compounds.
- Learn about food preparation methods, cooking techniques, and nutrient combinations that enhance absorption and utilization.
- Promote satiety by selecting whole, minimally processed foods and avoiding highly processed options.
- Consult a professional to evaluate your food log, make personalized recommendations, and ensure your nutritional choices align with your goals.
- Regular tracking of food intake, monitoring progress, and adjusting based on individual responses enable you to refine your nutrition plan over time.

You will achieve a better quality of life when all three domains are balanced. Of course, it often sounds easier than it is. The problem comes down to the bad habit of focusing on the superficial. We all want a quick fix, and improving your quality of life isn't so simple. Each Quality of Life Domain must be dissected and reconstructed. It is a process. However, each domain has concepts and principles guided by three tenets to make the journey more manageable. Let's explore the nine tenets before focusing on the concepts and principles under each domain.

Takeaways

- Your mind controls everything
- You cannot consistently change your actions until you fundamentally change your thoughts
- Improving your fitness will improve your ability to handle external stress
- Physical ability is the key to improving body confidence
- Making good nutrition choices increases food freedom
- Metabolic function, body composition, and reduced inflammation start with effective nutrition.

Resources

- Get **FREE** Bonus material that includes a complete breakdown and analysis of the most common fitness and nutrition programs to help you evaluate which ones will work best for you by following the F2 Method.
- Join **Coach Bronson's Body Confident Support Group** on Discord and meet more people who are improving themselves every day. https://discord.coachbronson.com
- Download the **FREE Body Confident Book Bonus Material** and Community information at https://bodyconfidentbook.com.

CHAPTER 6

THE NINE TENETS

"Health is not valued until sickness comes." ~ *Thomas Fuller*

Remember, for each domain, you have your guiding tenets. Many focus heavily on one or two tenets in Systems of Function and rarely address anything in Thought Processes. This is why you get stuck, frustrated, and have difficulty being consistent. You need all Nine Tenets of Health to fully realize your best life.

Let's start with the Thought Processes tenets.

Mindset Tenets

The Mindset Domain is about how you think and perceive yourself and the world around you. You must understand and adopt the three tenets that determine your thought processes.

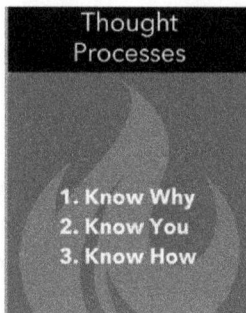

Image 6 - Tenets of Health 1-3

Mindset Tenet 1: Know Why You're Doing It

Define your Why and your Why Not. Understanding the reasons behind your actions is crucial for effective thought processes. This tenet emphasizes the importance of defining your *why* and *why not*. In other words, it's essential to identify the motivations and reasons that drive you toward a particular goal or decision and the reasons that might hinder your progress or prevent you from taking certain actions.

By clearly defining your motivations and potential obstacles, you gain a deeper understanding of your purpose and can make more informed choices.

Mindset Tenet 2: Know Who You Want to Be

Create a vision, establish an identity, and identify actions. This tenet focuses on self-awareness and personal development. It highlights the significance of creating a vision and establishing your desired identity. By envisioning who you want to become, you can align your actions and decisions with that vision. This reflective process involves identifying the actions, behaviors, and qualities that align with your desired identity.

By understanding who you want to be, you can make choices that align with your values and contribute to your personal growth.

Mindset Tenet 3: Know How You're Going to Get There

Set goals, make a plan, evaluate progress, and make adjustments. The third tenet focuses on the practical aspects of achieving your goals. It emphasizes the importance of setting clear goals, creating a plan, monitoring your progress, and making necessary adjustments along the way. Setting specific, measurable, attainable, relevant, and time-bound (SMART), goals provide you with a clear roadmap. Making a plan helps you break down your goals into manageable steps.

Regularly evaluating your progress allows you to identify what is working and what needs improvement. This process enables you to adjust, refine your approach, and stay on track toward your desired outcomes.

Applying the Mindset Tenet 1 Through 3

Scenario: Ken has consumed every bit of information he can about how to get in shape. He's learned about a dozen methods to build muscle and just as many different diet hacks to increase his metabolism and optimize his mitochondria.

None of it is working. He's at a complete loss. He keeps trying but is failing to make progress.

Tenet 1 - Know Your Why: Ken hasn't done the work to figure out why he wants to build muscle. He doesn't have an emotional connection to the driving force behind his motivation. Without a clear Why, Ken falls prey to interesting information and exciting new ideas and has no way to filter them against what he wants to achieve.

Tenet 2 - Know who you want to be: Because Ken doesn't have a strong Why, he's not been able to develop a picture of what he wants his life to look like or what will change when he reaches his goal. Without a vision of his future, he has nothing to guide his current actions that will drive him in the direction he needs to go.

Tenet 3 - Know how you will get there: Without a Why, it's impossible to set a goal or develop a plan for reaching it. A map is useless if you don't know where you're going.

Recommendations: Ken needs to figure out his real motivations and develop a vision for what he wants his life to look like when those things become a reality. Then he can start doing what he needs to do, set some goals, and follow a plan to stay consistent until he creates the life he wants.

Doing this will prevent constantly jumping from program to program and being confused about what new thing to try every other week.

These three Tenets of Health emphasize the importance of under-standing your motivations, envisioning your desired identity, and implementing practical strategies to achieve your goals. Following these tenets can enhance your critical thinking skills, support personal development, improve consistency, and build long-term success. When you have clarity in your thought process, you will more easily navigate your fitness and nutrition. Both have tenets to help guide you in their respective domains.

Fitness and Nutrition Tenets

While the mindset tenets fall under thought processes, the fitness and nutrition tenets are founded in the Systems of Function tenets. Your quality of life is reliant on how well your body functions. Referring back to the Wellness Continuum, we see that sickness is essentially dysfunction, and wellness is optimal function. The more you can improve how your body works, the better everything will be. So, let's dive into our Systems of Function tenets. We will start with the Fitness Domain and tenets four through six.

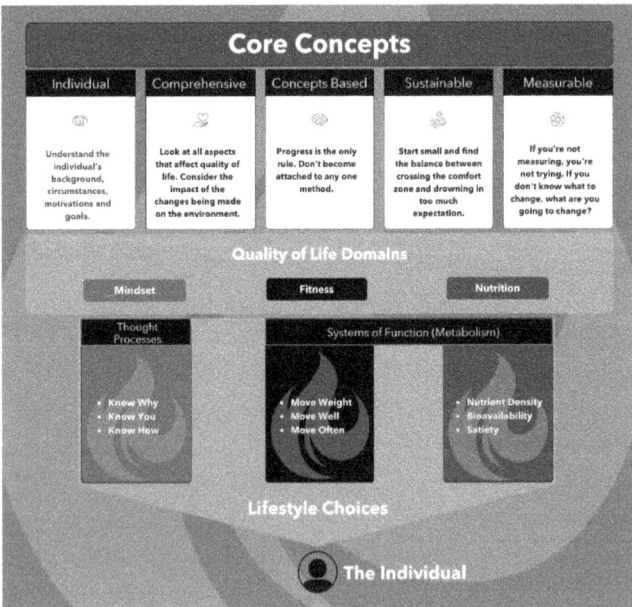

Core Concepts

Individual	Comprehensive	Concepts Based	Sustainable	Measurable
Understand the individual's background, circumstances, motivations and goals.	Look at all aspects that affect quality of life. Consider the impact of the changes being made on the environment.	Progress is the only rule. Don't become attached to any one method.	Start small and find the balance between crossing the comfort zone and drowning in too much expectation.	If you're not measuring, you're not trying. If you don't know what to change, what are you going to change?

Quality of Life Domains

Mindset	Fitness	Nutrition
Thought Processes	Systems of Function (Metabolism)	
• Know Why • Know You • Know How	• Move Weight • Move Well • Move Often	• Nutrient Density • Bioavailability • Satiety

Lifestyle Choices

The Individual

Image 7 - Tenets of Health 4-9

Fitness Tenet 4: Move Well

Understand the benefits and application of Technique, Consistency, and Intensity. This tenet emphasizes the importance of proper movement technique, consistency in training, and appropriate intensity levels.

By focusing on technique, you can perform exercises correctly, reducing the risk of injury and maximizing the effectiveness of your workouts. Consistency is critical for progress, as regular exercise over time leads to adaptation and improved fitness. Intensity refers to challenging the body appropriately to stimulate adaptations but without going beyond one's capabilities.

Finding the right technique, consistency, and intensity balance helps you optimize your fitness journey and achieve your desired goals.

Fitness Tenet 5: Move Weight

Muscles need stimulus; the body needs a challenge. Adaptation to increases in stress requires controlled increases in stress. This tenet recognizes that muscles require stimulation to grow and become stronger. By incorporating resistance training and gradually increasing the challenge or load placed on the muscles, you can promote muscle growth, improve strength, and enhance overall function.

Controlled increases in stress, such as gradually progressing in weight or resistance, allow the body to adapt and prevent overexertion or injury. Moving weight through traditional weightlifting or bodyweight exercises helps you build muscle, improve bone density, and support healthy body composition.

Fitness Tenet 6: Move Often

Adaptation and growth need consistency over time. Taking frequent breaks or constantly changing the program is counterproductive. Consistency in exercise is crucial for long-term improvements and optimal function. This tenet highlights the importance of incorporating regular physical activity into daily routines.

Consistent movement patterns allow the body to adapt and grow, improving cardiovascular fitness, muscular strength, and overall stamina. Taking frequent breaks or constantly changing exercise programs can disrupt progress and hinder adaptation. Moving often and maintaining consistency in physical activity supports your fitness goals and contributes to your overall well-being.

Applying The Fitness Tenets 4 through 6

Scenario: Zoey wants to build muscle and get stronger to do more outdoor activities with her grandchildren. She started lifting three days a week and really enjoys her time working out.

She's been having knee pain for a couple of weeks, and when she gets on her body composition scale, it's only showing minimal improvement in her muscle mass.

Tenet 4 - Move Well: Zoey likely has pain from improper movement in some exercises. There may have always been improper movement that was never a real issue because she was never doing enough activity for it to matter.

Tenet 5 - Move Weight: Is Zoey using enough weight or pushing herself to do enough reps to stimulate muscle growth? Muscles need adequate intensity and volume to start growing.

Tenet 6 - Move Often: Is she doing one body part per week or full body each time she works out? It sounds like Zoey is doing enough, but it's possible she could adjust her routine to allow for more intensity on fewer body parts by adding an additional day per week to her schedule.

Recommendation: First thing to do is get her knees looked at by a Physical Therapist and identify what's going on. Rehabilitation for any identified issues should be included in her training plan. Other movements should also be evaluated to ensure she can perform them consistently enough to add intensity as she progresses.

She should work with a trainer to evaluate how she's working out, educate her on how to pick appropriate weights and show her what proper intensity looks and feels like.

Based on those things, Zoey may want to add a day, or she might be good with her schedule based on her improved ability to apply what she's learned in every workout.

Of course, movement requires fuel, and your fuel comes from nutrition. The last three tenets fall under the Nutrition Domain. Nutrients matter the most—they are the reason we eat. A focus on nutrient density is a focus on optimal function. So, let's jump into the last three tenets under nutrition.

Nutrition Tenet 7: Nutrient Density

This tenet emphasizes the importance of prioritizing nutrient-dense foods in one's diet. Nutrient density refers to the concentration of essential vitamins, minerals, and other beneficial compounds in relation to the caloric content of a food.

Choosing foods rich in nutrients provides your body with the necessary building blocks for optimal function and overall health. Nutrient-dense foods support various physiological processes, including energy production, immune function, tissue repair, and cognitive function. Focusing on nutrient density ensures you nourish your bodies with high-quality fuel to support your well-being.

Nutrition Tenet 8: Bioavailability

If your body can't use it, the nutrition doesn't matter. Make choices that improve your chances of getting the most out of the food. Bioavailability refers to how nutrients from food are absorbed and utilized by the body. This tenet highlights the importance of considering factors that influence bioavailability, such as food preparation methods, cooking techniques, and combinations of nutrients.

Optimal bioavailability ensures that the body can effectively absorb and utilize the nutrients the diet provides. Making choices that enhance bioavailability, such as pairing certain nutrients together (e.g., combining vitamin C-rich foods with iron-rich foods for better iron absorption), can maximize the nutritional benefits obtained from the diet.

Nutrition Tenet 9: Satiety

Avoid *fake* food. Food has an impact on how your hormones and your brain react. Choose foods that are healthy for your body and your mind. Satiety refers to the feeling of fullness and satisfaction after a meal. This tenet highlights the importance of selecting whole, minimally processed foods that provide sustained energy, promote satiety, and support overall well-being.

Highly processed or *fake* foods, often high in added sugars, unhealthy fats, and artificial additives, can disrupt hormonal balance, lead to cravings, and negatively affect mental well-being. Choosing nutrient-dense, natural foods that nourish the body and mind promotes satiety, helps regulate appetite, and contributes to optimal function. When you put all nine tenets together, it looks like this:

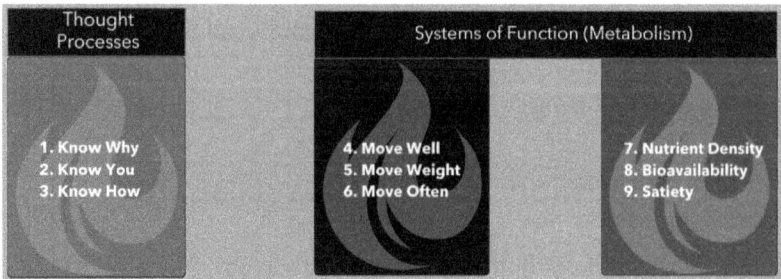

Thought Processes	Systems of Function (Metabolism)	
1. Know Why 2. Know You 3. Know How	4. Move Well 5. Move Weight 6. Move Often	7. Nutrient Density 8. Bioavailability 9. Satiety

Image 5 - Lifestyle Categories w/Tenets of Health

Applying the Nutrition Tenets 7 Through 9

Scenario: Bryce has everything locked down. He's got a solid workout routine, and his nutrition is on point. He feels great, and he hits his macros on the dime every day. Bryce likes to stay healthy but lean, with around sixteen to eighteen percent body fat. He's noticed that although his workouts are great, and he feels good, his body fat percentage is increasing. He's almost at twenty percent, and he's not sure what's going on.

Tenet 7 - Nutrient Density: When Bryce's coach looks at his food log, he notices Bryce is eating multiple protein shakes daily to meet his protein goals. Bryce also uses a lot of cream in his coffee in the morning. Both of these options are great for macros but poor for nutrients. Bryce is not providing his body with the micronutrients it needs to function.

Tenet 8 - Bioavailability: The rest of Bryce's food log looks pretty good. His coach notices that Bryce has grilled chicken breast salad daily with kale. Bryce's coach points out that kale can harm the bioavailability of other foods due to its high oxalate content.

Tenet 9 - Satiety: With Bryce getting a large portion of his macros from shakes and heavy cream, he has difficulty snacking between meals. Of course, he doesn't always track those times it happens. "It's not that often," he tells himself.

Recommendation: Eat more real food. Bryce is getting a lot of material into his system but not nearly enough nutrients. Some of the nutrients he does get aren't accessible to his body because other factors inhibit them.

If Bryce increased his red meat intake and maybe added some eggs to his coffee instead of heavy cream, he would raise his effectiveness in all three of the Nutrition Domain Tenets of Health.

Understanding and incorporating these tenets into daily routines, activities, and food choices can optimize your fitness, nutrition, and overall quality of life. These tenets and other aspects of the F2 Method provide a blueprint for approaching a well-rounded lifestyle that supports optimal function, well-being, and long-term success. With that, it is crucial to understand that this is a blueprint—a guide.

Remember when I said to follow concepts, not rules? Let's get into the concepts and principles!

Takeaways

- You must have a why and/or a why not. Your emotional connection to the end result is the only thing that will keep you on track over time.
- Stop eating fake food. Labels are only put on consumable that offer less than nutritious value.
- Macros are important but they don't equal nutrition.
- Fitness requires discomfort.
- Consistent effort beats intensity every time. Just get started and don't stop.

Resources

- Get **FREE** Bonus material that includes a complete breakdown and analysis of the most common fitness and nutrition programs to help you evaluate which ones will work best for you by following the F2 Method.
- Join **Coach Bronson's Body Confident Support Group** on Discord and meet more people who are improving themselves every day. https://discord.coachbronson.com
- Download the **FREE Body Confident Book Bonus Material** and Community information at https://bodyconfidentbook.com.

CHAPTER 7

- -

MINDSET DOMAIN CONCEPTS AND PRINCIPLES

"To create something exceptional, your mindset must be relentlessly focused on the smallest detail."
~ Giorgio Armani

I f there is any part of this book you absolutely need to read, this is it. How you think about yourself, the work you have to do, and your challenges determine how arduous the journey is and how much success you will have.

The process of changing how you think takes time. I often see people who are *stalled* and think it's because of something wrong with their bodies or because they aren't doing something correctly. In many cases, a shift in their thoughts and beliefs gets them unstuck and moving again. Mindset shifts require us to develop self-awareness and a willingness to think and do things differently than we're used to.

Resistance to change is often an indicator that change needs to happen.

Identifying with a thought process, "I'm not a gym person;" or "I'm an all-or-nothing kind of person," is the fastest way to limit your potential.

> *How you've done things up to now has gotten you to this point. It cannot get you anywhere else.*

There are eleven different thought paradigms you need to understand and apply to your life. You will probably never master all of them. You can, however, learn them, understand them, and do your best to practice them every chance you get.

The cool thing is, now you have a reference you can go back to if you ever need a reminder.

Eleven Thought Paradigms

- **It's Up to You:** This principle underscores the importance of personal responsibility and self-agency. You are the ultimate master of your destiny, and your choices, actions, and mindset all contribute to the outcomes in your life.

- **You Need a Why and a Why Not:** You should have a clear reason for why you want to achieve something (the 'why') and why you wouldn't want the opposite to happen (the 'why not'). These factors help to motivate and steer you toward your goals.

- **Setting Goals:** This principle refers to identifying what you want to achieve and establishing measurable goals and time frames. The process helps provide direction, structure, and a roadmap for success.

- **The Truth About Motivation:** Understanding motivation involves recognizing what it is. It's essential to develop an honest assessment of what you want and what you're willing to do to get it.

- **What is Consistency:** Consistency is the key to progress. It's not about perfection but persistently doing the necessary tasks over time, even when difficult.

- **Why You Need Grit:** Grit is the combination of passion and perseverance. It helps you to stick with your goals, especially during challenging times. Grit can be a better predictor of success than talent or IQ.

- **Embrace the Boring:** Not all tasks on the road to success will be exciting. This principle encourages embracing repetitive or mundane tasks as they often form the foundation for achievement.
- **The Rest of Your Life:** This highlights the importance of long-term thinking and sustainability. Any changes made should be ones you can maintain throughout your life, not just short-term fixes.
- **Apply Context and Perspective:** This refers to viewing situations within their larger context and from various angles. It encourages reframing challenges as opportunities for growth and learning.
- **If You're Not Tracking, You're Not Trying:** This principle advocates for tracking progress to stay accountable, maintain focus, and assess what's working or not working.
- **Avoid Extremes. Make Adjustments, not Swings:** This principle suggests making smaller, incremental adjustments rather than making drastic changes or following extreme measures. This allows for sustainable change and reduces the risk of burnout or reversal.

Are you ready, willing, and able to think differently? I hope so. It will make the process of change a lot easier and more fulfilling. However, it is all up to you!

It's Up to You

Taking personal responsibility and ownership means acknowledging your role in your life: the choices you make, the actions you take, and the consequences of those actions. It involves understanding that you are the primary agent in shaping your life and accepting accountability for your decisions, successes, and failures.

No one is coming to rescue you.

Personal responsibility and ownership manifest in several ways:

- **Making Decisions:** This is about recognizing that you control your decisions. Whether it's your career, personal relationships, or lifestyle, the decisions you make directly impact the course of your life.
- **Facing the consequences:** Taking personal responsibility means accepting the outcomes of your actions, both positive and negative. Instead of blaming others or external circumstances, you acknowledge that your choices led to the situation.
- **Learning and Growing:** With personal responsibility, you see mistakes and setbacks as opportunities for learning and growth rather than defining failures. This enables personal and professional development.
- **Taking the Initiative:** This involves being proactive and taking steps to improve your life instead of waiting for things to happen or for others to do something for you.

The benefits of personal responsibility and ownership are:

- **Empowerment:** When you take responsibility for your actions, you assert control over your life. This sense of empowerment can boost your self-confidence and motivate you to pursue your goals.
- **Problem-Solving Skills:** By owning your decisions and consequences, you will likely develop strong problem-solving skills. You'll better identify potential problems, develop solutions, and make informed decisions.
- **Trust and Respect:** Taking responsibility can also earn you the trust and respect of others. People are more likely to respect and trust someone who holds themselves accountable and owns up to their mistakes.
- **Personal Growth:** Accepting personal responsibility can foster personal growth. By facing challenges head-on and learning from your mistakes, you gain wisdom, resilience, and a greater understanding of yourself.

Taking personal responsibility is a vital part of personal development and success. It fosters a proactive mindset, increases resilience, improves problem-solving skills, and can significantly improve your personal and professional relationships.

Your role as the primary change agent in your life cannot be over-stated. It is you who holds the power to bring about transformation in your thoughts, actions, and overall life. No matter how many self-help books you read or life coaches you consult, unless you decide to take action to alter your thoughts and perspectives, the change you desire will remain a far-off dream.

Understanding this is crucial. You are the architect of your own life. The power of your actions and decisions cannot be underestimated. The concept of "It's up to you," is about acknowledging this power and taking responsibility for it.

It's about making a commitment to yourself and sticking to it. When you decide to change, grow, and evolve, you will start noticing a difference.

Don't wait for circumstances to change, don't wait for others to make the first move. Take that step today. Because ultimately, it's up to you.

You Need a Why and a Why Not

Why do you want to change? What are you afraid of? What don't you want in your life anymore? What could your life look like?

Your Why represents the purpose or the reason behind your actions, decisions, or goals. It gives you direction and helps you understand what is important to you. This can help to guide your efforts and keep you focused when distractions or challenges arise.

When you know your why, you have a deeper level of motivation. This is because you're not just working towards a goal or action for the sake of it but because it aligns with your values or desired outcomes. This internal motivation can sustain you when external motivation may wane.

Knowing your why helps you to push through difficulties and maintain resilience. When confronted with challenges or setbacks, remembering your why can give you the strength to continue because you understand the larger purpose or goal you are striving towards.

Your Why Not is the set of reasons or factors that drive you to avoid specific outcomes or scenarios in your life. This may be fueled by fears, undesirable circumstances, or past experiences you do not wish to repeat. In essence, your why not is the flip side of your why. It represents what you are working against rather than what you are working toward.

Fear, while often seen as a negative emotion, can sometimes be a powerful motivator. For instance, the fear of poor health might motivate someone to eat better and exercise regularly. In this case, the why not is the fear of illness or disease.

Your why not could be tied to avoiding scenarios you don't want in your life. For example, if you grew up in a financially unstable home, your why not might be the desire to avoid similar financial instability in your own life.

Past experiences, particularly mistakes or failures, can shape your why not. For example, if a previous career choice led to dissatisfaction or burnout, your why not may involve avoiding a similar career path.

Your **Why** and **Why Not** are the source of your desire to reach your goals. Here's the kicker. They must be emotionally driven, or the temptation and emotional triggers you're trying to change will override them when things get rough.

Finding your deep-rooted emotional desire takes time, patience, honesty, and a willingness to confront and address painful issues. If you're willing to do that, you will find a level of drive you never knew you had.

Setting Goals

Your Why will give you the drive and motivation to work hard. You still need to know what you're working for and where you're going. Goals give you a direction to aim for and can help you maintain focus on your priorities.

Without them, you might drift aimlessly without making meaningful progress in any specific area. Goals help you effectively channel your energy and resources toward achieving desired outcomes. They give you a way to track and gauge your progress.

Be S.M.A.R.T

To make sure your goals are clear and reachable, each one should be

- **S**pecific (simple, sensible, significant).
- **M**easurable (meaningful, motivating).
- **A**chievable (agreed, attainable).
- **R**elevant (reasonable, realistic and resourced, results-based).
- **T**ime-bound (time-based, time-limited, time/cost limited, timely, time-sensitive).

S.M.A.R.T. goals require you to define precisely what you want to achieve. This clarity removes ambiguity and provides a clear direction for your efforts. Instead of having a vague goal like "get fit," a specific goal would be "run a 5K in under thirty minutes."

SPECIFIC: Your goal should be clear and specific. Otherwise, you won't focus your efforts or feel truly motivated to achieve it. When drafting your goal, try to answer the five "W" questions:

- What do I want to accomplish?
- Why is this goal important?
- Who is involved?
- Which resources or limits are involved?

For example: I want to build muscle mass and improve my strength.

MEASURABLE: Having measurable goals to track your progress and stay motivated is essential. Assessing progress helps you stay focused, meet your deadlines, and feel the excitement of getting closer to achieving your goal. How will you know when you've reached the goal? A measurable goal should address questions such as:

- How much?
- How long?
- How fast?
- How heavy?

For example: I want to build five pounds of muscle mass and improve my strength to squat my body weight one time.

ACHIEVABLE: Your goal must also be realistic and attainable to succeed. In other words, it should stretch your abilities but remain possible. When you set an achievable goal, you may identify previously overlooked opportunities or resources that can bring you closer to it. An attainable goal will usually answer questions such as:

- How can I accomplish this goal?
- How realistic is the goal, based on other constraints, finances, or work schedule?

For example: I want to build five pounds of muscle mass and improve my strength to squat my body weight one time. I will do this by resistance training three times a week and eating one time my lean body mass in grams of protein daily.

Tip: Make sure you are setting goals for yourself. Don't be persuaded into saying you want to accomplish something just to make someone else happy or fulfill what you think someone else's desire for you is. Find out what excites you about your new life and go in that direction.

RELEVANT: This step ensures that your goal matters to you and aligns with other relevant goals. We all need support and assistance in achieving our goals, but it's crucial to retain control over them. So, ensure that your plans drive everyone forward but that you're still responsible for achieving your goal. A relevant goal can answer "yes" to these questions:

- Does this seem worthwhile?
- Will this goal have a positive impact on my life?
- Does this match other efforts/needs?

For example: I want to build five pounds of muscle mass and improve my strength to squat my body weight one time. I will do this by resistance training three times a week and eating one time my lean body mass in grams of protein per day. Doing this will improve my daily energy and reduce my back pain.

TIME-BOUND: Every goal needs a target date, a deadline to focus on, and something to work toward. This part of the SMART goals criteria prevents everyday tasks from taking priority over your longer-term goals. A time-bound goal will usually answer these questions:

- When?
- What can I do six months from now?
- What can I do six weeks from now?
- What can I do today?

For example: In the next six months, I want to build five pounds of muscle mass and improve my strength to squat my body weight one time. I will do this by resistance training three times a week and eating one time my lean body mass in grams of protein daily. Doing this will improve my daily energy and reduce my back pain.

Now that's a goal you can build a solid plan from. What will your first goal be?

The Truth About Motivation

You're not lacking motivation. You don't need to be motivated. You just have to decide if you really want it or not.

Motivation is a representation of desire or wanting something. It's an internal drive that propels you to take action and pursue a certain goal or outcome. Because of its inherent nature, motivation cannot be handed to you by another person, like a physical object. It is not a feeling that you can switch on and off. Instead, it arises from within you, stemming from your interests, aspirations, and needs.

If you're motivated, you want it enough to do the work. If you're not motivated, you don't want it enough to do the work.

If you're genuinely motivated to achieve something, it means that you truly want it. You are willing to invest effort, overcome challenges, and make sacrifices to reach that goal. Conversely, lacking motivation toward a particular goal may indicate that you do not value or desire it strongly enough.

The balance between the desire for something new and the resistance to change or loss. Let's unpack these two components:

- **The Desire for Something New:** This is the driving force that propels you toward a goal or an outcome. It's a craving for an improved situation, a new skill, a promotion, better health, etc. The intensity of this desire often reflects the perceived value of the goal – the greater the perceived benefits or rewards, the stronger the desire.

- **Resistance to Change or Loss:** This is the force that pulls you back or hinders you from pursuing a goal. It could arise from fear of the unknown, fear of failure, complacency, or the perceived costs of pursuing the goal, including effort, time, or the loss of comfort or security. The intensity of resistance often correlates with the perceived risks or drawbacks of the change.

These two forces are in constant interplay, forming a balance that influences your level of motivation. To feel motivated to pursue a goal, the desire for the new thing or the perceived benefits of change must outweigh the resistance or perceived costs. You feel motivated to act when the scale tips in favor of desire.

For instance, consider a person who wants to start a fitness routine. Their desire might be fueled by wanting better health, improved self-esteem, or increased energy levels. However, they might resist due to factors like the effort required, fear of injury, loss of leisure time, or the comfort of their current routine. If the desire for the benefits of exercise outweighs the resistance, they will be motivated to start and maintain a fitness routine.

However, it's crucial to note that this balance is not static; it can shift over time due to changes in circumstances, perceived benefits and costs, or emotional states. Therefore, regularly reassessing your desires and resistances can be crucial to maintaining or enhancing motivation.

> *Your level of motivation directly results from the depth and emotional connection you have to your Why and Why Not.*

Ultimately, motivation comes down to understanding yourself—what you want, why, and how much you're willing to do to achieve it. It's a call to personal responsibility, prompting you to be the active agent in your life, setting and pursuing your goals based on your desires and values. It highlights the importance of self-reflection, self-awareness, and self-direction in living a fulfilling and meaningful life.

What is Consistency?

Consistency is a fundamental principle of progress, not a benchmark of perfection. It is about making incremental progress over time, often by making more positive than negative choices. Conversely, perfection sets an unattainable standard that often leads to disappointment, stress, and feelings of inadequacy.

Let's take an example. Suppose you're trying to adopt a healthier lifestyle. Perfection would demand that you eat a flawless diet, work out every single day, never indulge in junk food, and always get the perfect amount of sleep. But realistically, this is an incredibly tough, if not impossible, standard to maintain. You're likely to falter somewhere; when you do, the perfectionist mindset often leads to feelings of failure.

On the contrary, consistency in this context would mean making healthier choices more often than not: choosing the bun-less burger most of the time, working out regularly, allowing yourself rest days, and enjoying an occasional healthy treat. Here, you don't beat yourself up when you have a bad day or miss a day of exercise because the focus is not on never making mistakes but on making more positive choices than negative ones over time.

The key is understanding that it's okay to stumble. Everyone does. It's not about never falling but getting up each time you fall. Failure isn't just inevitable; it's necessary. Every time you fail, you learn something new. You understand better what doesn't work, which helps guide you toward what does.

Embracing failure as a learning opportunity rather than a dead end is a much healthier and more effective mindset for achieving your goals.

It allows you to treat mistakes as stepping stones rather than stumbling blocks. This is often called a **Growth Mindset:** the belief that abilities and understanding can be developed with time and effort.

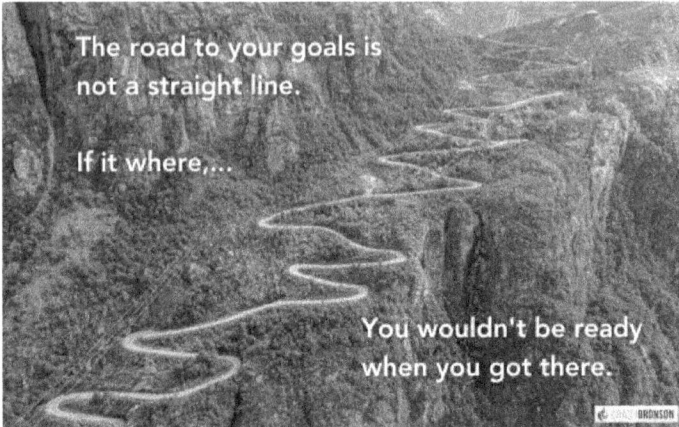

The road to your goals is not a straight line.

If it where,...

You wouldn't be ready when you got there.

Remember, the journey towards any goal is never a straight path; it's a winding road filled with ups and downs. And that's okay. It's those twists and turns that make the journey interesting and rewarding. So, focus on being consistent, not perfect. Consistency is a kinder, more forgiving approach to reaching your goals. It values effort, recognizes progress, and understands that every step you take, no matter how small, is a step in the right direction.

The Secret to Staying Consistent

Start thinking in terms of NET Positive and NET Negative Impact. I like this better than weighing the Pros and Cons. With Pros and Cons, the focus tends to be on you and what you're feeling, what you like or don't like. It can be a challenge to separate from the emotion of the moment.

The concept of NET Impact completely removes you from the equation. A NET Impact evaluation compares the choice to the desired result, not how you feel about the choice.

A NET Positive is less likely to be related to your feelings. A NET Negative is more likely to be related to your goal.

Scenario: At a party, someone offers you a glass of wine.

In a Pro vs. Con comparison, you would justify the wine with things like:

- It's only one glass, and I've been good this week.
- I don't want to be rude; I'm just being polite.
- I've been stressed lately, and this will help me relax.

The Cons are still compelling but aren't tied to your Why, Why Not, or your Goals:

- I'll have a hangover tomorrow.
- I will have a crappy workout tomorrow if I even go.
- My sleep will be messed up for a few days.
- It will give me digestive issues this week.

To be more consistent, you must consider the process an investment. Then the scope and choices become more apparent.

The NET Positive impact of drinking a glass of wine compared to your fear of losing control of your health and being unable to break habits that will keep you from being self-reliant as you age. **ZERO.**

The NET Positive impact of drinking a glass of wine compared to your goal of losing five percent body fat and building two to five pounds of lean mass in the next six months. **ZERO.**

The NET Positive impact of drinking a glass of wine compared to your goal of reducing inflammation and maintaining good brain health as you get older. **ZERO.**

The NET Negative impact of drinking a glass of wine is obvious at this point. If there is no NET Positive, then abstinence is the only choice that moves you in the right direction.

Remember: **The Only Rule is Your Progress**

This kind of evaluation forces you to focus on things outside your emotional triggers. You will find that the more you base your decisions on the Reason and the Result, the easier it becomes to stay consistent.

Finally, take heed that consistency can be boring.

Embrace the Boring

Imagine this. You can be entirely free from medication, exhibit no metabolic issues, possess an ideal body composition, and rank within the top five percent of the world's fittest people. The catch? Your lifestyle must consist of consuming the same three foods every day and repeating the same fitness routine three times a week for the rest of your life. Could you commit to it? Could you handle the monotony?

Achievement hinges on your ability to embrace and excel in the basics—the mundane—which serve as the foundations of your Functional Systems. Straying from the essentials compromises your body's needs and sets you on a path away from your goals. We find success in routine—in what some might call *the boring stuff.*

Top-tier personal trainers often struggle to build their businesses, not due to lack of skill but because most people shun *boring* workouts. Yet, these seemingly dull routines consistently yield better results than their more complex or trendy counterparts.

Have you ever heard of the 10,000-hour rule? It's the concept that around 10,000 hours of practice are needed to master a skill. What if the skill was the art of living your best life? With approximately 5,800 waking hours in a year, how much time are you willing to dedicate to mastering the fundamentals until they are second nature?

Beware of the pitfalls of variety and shortcuts. Often, we are tempted by flashy novelties: an intriguing supplement, a revolutionary device, a novel metabolic protocol, or a groundbreaking exercise. These enticing solutions are distractions, promising an end to all our woes.

Indeed, consistency may not be glamorous, but it's a prerequisite for attaining and maintaining health and fitness. **The more boring it is, the more likely it will work.**

Embracing the boring isn't easy. It's well—boring. To endure the boring takes grit. But what does that mean, and do you really need it?

Grit: What Is It and Why You Need It

Grit is a psychological term that refers to a person's passion for a long-term goal and the powerful motivation to achieve that objective. Other words for grit are:

- Tenacity
- Perseverance
- Resolve
- Drive
- Purpose
- Determination
- Fortitude
- Stamina

Grit is a firmness of character and involves maintaining effort and interest over the years despite failures, adversity, and plateaus in progress. Grit has two key components:

- **Consistency of interest:** This is about having an enduring passion for the long-term goals or missions that provide meaning and purpose in life.
- **Perseverance of effort:** This refers to hard work and resilience in the face of setbacks, challenges, and failures.

So, how does grit help maintain consistency during challenges?

Grit is a resilience and perseverance toolkit. When faced with a challenge or a roadblock, perseverance keeps you pushing forward. It's what helps you keep going when the going gets tough. It's the mental toughness to face failure and to keep striving despite it. It's the commitment to keep working, even when you're tired, discouraged, or tempted to give up.

With this mental fortitude, you're not deterred by the effort the journey toward your goals may take. **You're not looking for the easy way out or the quick fix.** You're prepared to keep putting in the work, day after day, because you know that's what it takes to achieve your goal.

In the face of challenges, a gritty person maintains consistency by not allowing setbacks to deter them from their path. They understand that progress isn't always linear and that setbacks are an inevitable part of any journey. Instead of being discouraged by these challenges, they use them as learning opportunities and motivation to push harder and keep going.

In this way, grit can help you maintain consistency in facing challenges. It gives you the resilience to keep making positive choices and taking positive actions towards your goals, even when it's hard, even when you fail, and even when progress seems slow or non-existent. It's about playing the long game and recognizing that setbacks are just part of the process, not the end of the road.

Grit isn't just about brute force, though. It also involves being adaptable and flexible, knowing when to pivot or take a different approach, and continually learning and adjusting along the way. It's about staying committed to your goals but being flexible in your approach to achieving them.

The plan may change, but the goal remains the same.

Tenacity is critical in achieving long-term goals and is considered a key ingredient to success and fulfillment in various areas of life, including education, career, health, and relationships. Here's why you need it:

- **Persistence Through Challenges:** Life is inevitably filled with obstacles and setbacks. Whether it's a difficult project at work, a demanding course at school, or a personal goal that's taking longer to achieve than you'd hoped, grit can keep you going. Grit allows you to persist even when you face difficulties and is essential for maintaining momentum during challenging times.
- **Achieving Long-Term Goals:** Success in almost any field requires a long-term commitment. Grit enables you to maintain focus and passion over the long haul, not just for days or weeks, but for years. This sustained effort and consistency can often be the difference between achieving your goals or falling short.
- **Resilience:** Grit strengthens your resilience, the ability to recover from setbacks, adapt to change, and keep going in the face of adversity. Resilience is a critical life skill that helps you deal with daily stressors and significant life events.
- **Personal Growth:** Grit can foster personal growth because it often involves learning from mistakes and failures. Instead of

giving up after a setback, people with grit analyze what went wrong, learn from the experience, and use that knowledge to move forward.

- **Success and Fulfillment:** Research has shown that grit better predicts success than IQ or talent. While intelligence and talent are essential, benefits can be lost without the perseverance to apply them consistently over time. Intelligence and IQ do not guarantee outcomes because consistency of effort and perseverance of effort are often lacking. People tend to achieve goals and find greater fulfillment in accomplishments because they've put in the hard work and overcome the challenges along the way.

Tenacity, perseverance, purpose, fortitude—GRIT—is essential because it equips you to face challenges head-on, learn from your mistakes, and persist until you reach your goals in a complex and fast-paced world. We often assume that this character trait is something we are born with. However, you can develop it.

Developing grit involves nurturing a combination of passion, resilience, determination, and focus. Here are some strategies you can use:

- **Cultivate a Growth Mindset:** A growth mindset is a belief that you can develop your abilities and intelligence over time with effort, learning, and persistence. By embracing a growth mindset, you'll be more open to challenges, unafraid of making mistakes, and better equipped to learn from them, which fosters grit.
- **Find Your Why and Why Not:** Your reason for making change is a core component of perseverance. Spend time exploring what drives you and what emotional connections you have to the life you want to live. When genuinely interested and passionate about something, you are more likely to stick with it over the long term.
- **Set Long-term Goals:** Having clear and meaningful long-term goals can help cultivate your fortitude. When you know what you're working toward, it becomes easier to maintain the drive to persist and overcome challenges.

- **Embrace Challenges and Failures:** Don't fear setbacks and failures; they are integral to learning and growth. Each setback is a learning opportunity that brings you one step closer to your goal.
- **Practice Perseverance:** Practice sticking with tasks even when challenging or tedious. Start with small tasks to build your perseverance muscles.
- **Develop a Routine or Habit:** Consistent habits can help maintain the effort required to reach long-term goals. It could be as simple as dedicating a set number of hours each week to work on a specific skill or task.
- **Surround Yourself with Like-Minded People:** You are influenced by the people around you. Being around gritty people can inspire you to be more persistent and resilient.

Developing grit is not an overnight process. It requires time, patience, and dedication. But the effort can pay off in greater resilience, determination, and success in achieving your long-term goals. Part of this long-term process will require you to keep track of your progress.

If You're Not Tracking, You're Not Trying

There are two sides to the discussion about tracking. One side is the practical impact that tracking has on your progress and ability to adjust and improve your plan. The other is the mental aspect of your willingness to commit and adhere to that plan.

If only I had a penny for every time I heard someone say, "I hate tracking."

That's why I say, "If you're not tracking, you're not trying."

I want to impress upon you the importance of self-accountability and active involvement in your health and wellness journey. Making an effort to record, monitor, and evaluate your progress shows a high level of commitment and dedication to achieving your goals. The act of monitoring progress can help keep you motivated. Seeing tangible evidence of your progress can be a powerful incentive to continue working toward your goals. In contrast, if you're not seeing progress or regressing, it can be a wake-up call to reconsider your approach.

Tracking helps you become more aware of your habits and behaviors. This awareness is vital to making meaningful and lasting changes. If you're not tracking, it's easy to overlook or forget about unproductive behaviors, making it harder to address them. For example, you might notice that when you consume a particular type of food, you feel lethargic the next day, or after a specific exercise, you feel more energetic. Identifying these patterns can inform your decisions and lead to more effective strategies for improving your health.

Tracking is the only way to accurately determine what's working and what isn't. By recording your progress, you have the data necessary to make informed decisions about what adjustments might be needed to your diet, exercise routine, or lifestyle habits. Without this data, it's difficult to attribute changes in your health to specific adjustments you've made.

The practice of tracking encourages consistency, which is crucial to making progress toward health and wellness goals. Tracking can help to turn positive behaviors into regular habits. The act of recording encourages commitment to the habit and increases your mindfulness about it. Studies have even shown that we are better at committing information to memory when we write it down.

If you're not tracking, you may be more likely to put your health and wellness in the hands of others, relying on external opinions or generalized advice. Tracking encourages you to take ownership of your health and wellness journey, focusing on your unique needs and responses.

The beauty of recording your journey is that it can be as detailed or as simple as you need it to be. If you have the time and energy, you might track more rigorously, such as weighing every bit of food you eat. If you're pressed for time or find that level of detail overwhelming, you might opt for a more straightforward method, like taking pictures of your meals or keeping a food diary. The key is to make tracking manageable and sustainable while providing data that helps you make effective decisions.

What to Track

There are two things you can track. You can record the effort and actions you put into the process and track the results of those actions (input/output).

- **Tracking Actions/Effort (Input):** This refers to the active measures you take to achieve your goals. For health and fitness, this could include a wide range of things such as the frequency, intensity, and duration of your workouts, the types and quantities of food you're eating, hours of sleep per night, and even tracking psychological factors like stress levels or mood states. Essentially, you're monitoring your behavior and habits, which is valuable because it allows you to identify which actions contribute to your success and which may be holding you back.
- **Tracking Results (Output):** This is the measurable impact or outcome of your actions. For health and fitness, common examples could be body weight, body fat percentage, lean muscle mass, cardiovascular fitness, blood pressure, or other health markers like blood sugar levels. Tracking results is crucial because it shows the tangible effects of your efforts and allows you to see if you're moving toward your goal. It helps to validate that your actions are working, or alternatively, signals that something needs to be adjusted if you're not seeing the expected progress.

Things you can track are (not a comprehensive list):

- Strength
- Body Fat Percentage
- Number of days worked out
- Lean Mass
- How many hours of sleep
- Triglyceride to HDL Ratio
- Flexibility
- Macros
- Fasting Blood Sugar

- Inflammation Markers
- Repetitions of an Exercise
- Electrolyte intake
- Resting Heart Rate
- Self Care activities in a week
- Food choices
- Speed of a movement
- And so on

While tracking your actions and results is essential, the balance between them depends on your goals, the stage of your journey, and your personal preference. Some people may benefit more from focusing on the process, as it cultivates consistent habits and behaviors that lead to long-term success. Others may find motivation in monitoring results closely, using that data as a feedback loop to adjust their actions.

Remember that tracking isn't about perfection, and it's not meant to make you feel guilty or obsessive about every detail. Instead, it's about providing insights, understanding trends, and helping you make more informed choices that contribute to your overall health and wellness. With that, you might begin to notice some trends. These are important.

The Importance of Trends

I often have a "talking off the ledge" conversation with clients new to tracking. A common mistake people make is getting hung up on the numbers of any given measurement without looking at it in the context of everything else. They often think in terms of immediate results, not long-term progress.

This is where the overlap in concepts impacts your perspective. If you accept that your journey is lifelong, you are less inclined to get upset over one measurement in time. The process of evaluating data has to include sufficient time to determine the overall effect of changes you are making. The importance of analyzing trends over "point-in-time" data when measuring progress lies in the broader, more comprehensive perspective that trends provide. Here's why:

- **Variability:** In our daily lives, many factors can cause temporary fluctuations in our health and fitness data. For example, a single weigh-in could be affected by the amount of water you've consumed that day, hormonal changes, or even whether you've recently used the restroom. If you focus too heavily on point-in-time data, you may become disheartened by normal variations that aren't indicative of your overall progress.
- **Consistency:** Trends help you assess the consistency of your efforts over time. Consistent behavior is often the key to long-term success in health and fitness, so looking at trends can help you see if you are maintaining your habits over extended periods.
- **Patterns:** Trends can reveal patterns that point-in-time data can't. For example, if you track your fuel macro intake and weight over a month, you might see a pattern where higher-fuel days lead to temporary weight increases. Still, overall, your weight is trending downward because your fuel intake is balanced.
- **Progress Over Time:** Perhaps the most significant benefit of examining trends is seeing your progress over time. A single point-in-time data can only tell you your status at a specific moment, but a trend can show you how far you've come. This information is crucial in fitness and health, where changes often occur gradually and can be hard to notice in the short term.
- **Predict Future Outcomes:** Trends also allow you to predict future outcomes. By understanding how you've progressed so far, you can estimate future progress, assuming similar conditions and efforts continue.

While point-in-time data can be helpful in certain short-term evaluations, focusing on trends is much more beneficial when measuring long-term progress and making sustainable health and fitness decisions. Emphasizing trends over single data points is crucial as it provides a more accurate picture of your progress, filtering out daily fluctuations and highlighting long-term change. This comprehensive approach to tracking aids in understanding your journey better, making informed decisions, and maintaining consistent motivation.

Consistency and tracking will also help you avoid the extremes.

Avoid Extremes, Make Adjustments Not Swings

The easiest way I can tell if someone has a short-term, fast-results mindset is by looking at their extreme choices. I regularly see people jumping from one direction to another with little to no time or objective evaluation of what's working or why.

Sudden, drastic changes are not sustainable in the long term and can potentially cause strain on your body and mind. Instead, focus on small, gradual adjustments that align with your personal goals and lifestyle. This way, you'll be better equipped to incorporate these changes into your routine, leading to consistent and sustainable progress.

Examples of what **not** to do:

- Focus on high fat intake for six months, realize it's not helping you lose weight, then go very low fat with high protein to see if that works.
- Go from not doing any fitness activity to having a goal to reach 10,000 steps a day, work out five days a week, and do thirty minutes of cardio every day.
- Decide that you'll go Keto, intermittent fast, get twenty minutes of sunlight every day, and go to bed an hour earlier every night— all simultaneously.

The more extreme the change, the less likely you are to maintain it.
Examples of what **to** do:

- Adjust your fat or protein goal by no more than five to ten grams per day, and wait at least four to six weeks before you adjust it again.
- Go from not doing any fitness activity to setting a goal to do some kind of movement for at least fifteen minutes three to four days a week.
- Decide to change your nutrition habits by removing French fries from your diet.

Remember that the goal is to improve your quality of life. Big swings in your routine usually increase stress and make things more complicated. That's the opposite of what you're trying to do. If it's causing more negative pressure, it's probably not sustainable. You have to maintain what you're doing to keep what you're getting. The results you're currently enjoying are a product of the consistent efforts you've been putting in. To preserve these results or to continue seeing progress, you need to continue those behaviors.

Let's say you've achieved your fitness goal by following a specific exercise routine and nutritional plan. Once you've reached that goal, it doesn't mean you can stop those practices and expect to maintain the results. Instead, you must continue with your routine and diet to sustain the progress you've made. Your previous issues (like weight gain, muscle loss, or low energy) may reappear if you revert to old habits.

Of course, adjustments and changes might be necessary over time due to evolving goals, body adaptations, or lifestyle changes. But the principle remains the same: the behaviors that got you to a healthier place are typically those needed to keep you there.

Drastic changes can significantly impact your mental state, biology, physiology, and neurology. Here's how:

- **Mental State:** Sudden, significant changes can trigger stress, anxiety, and feelings of being overwhelmed. This can be due to the discomfort of breaking away from familiar routines or the fear of failing to meet the new, more demanding standards you've set for yourself. If these feelings persist, it could lead to burnout or a lack of motivation to continue your health and fitness journey.
- **Biology:** Drastic dietary changes can disrupt your body's metabolic balance. For instance, suddenly switching to a highly restrictive diet may lead to nutrient deficiencies, impact hormone balance, or negatively affect gut health. Stress can increase cortisol, the stress hormone. Cortisol can create biological havoc.
- **Physiology:** When it comes to physical activity, sudden increases in intensity or duration can increase the risk of injuries, muscle strain, and exhaustion. Additionally, your body may not have the time to adapt to the new physical demands, which can impede progress in the long run.

- **Neurology:** Sudden changes can disrupt established neurological pathways, making new habits harder to adopt and maintain. Over time, this can result in a pattern of starting and stopping new routines, which may discourage you from making positive changes.

Implementing gradual changes that allow your mind and body to adapt over time is often more beneficial and sustainable than drastically altering your lifestyle. The smaller the changes are, the more likely you are to be consistent. You have a better chance of understanding your impact, and if you need to step back, it's less of a disruption to the plan.

Now, let's talk about fitness.

Takeaways

- No one can do this for you. Unless you take ownership of your journey, you will be at the mercy of your emotions and constantly trying things that don't work.
- You can't receive motivation. You create it by staying in touch with your emotional desire to succeed.
- Either you want it or you don't . The actions you take will tell you which one is driving you.
- Tracking doesn't have to be overwhelimg or forever.
- If you aren't tracking you can't make changes with any certain expectation of success.

Resources

- Get **FREE** Bonus material that includes a complete breakdown and analysis of the most common fitness and nutrition programs to help you evaluate which ones will work best for you by following the F2 Method.
- Join **Coach Bronson's Body Confident Support Group** on Discord and meet more people who are improving themselves every day. https://discord.coachbronson.com
- Download the **FREE Body Confident Book Bonus Material** and Community information at https://bodyconfidentbook.com.

CHAPTER 8

FITNESS DOMAIN CONCEPTS AND PRINCIPLES

"Take care of your body. It's the only place you have to live." ~ Jim Rohn

---

Fitness is a multifaceted concept, with principles encompassing various aspects of physical well-being and overall health. It plays a crucial role in enhancing your quality of life by improving physical performance, reducing the risk of disease, and promoting mental and emotional well-being. To fully understand fitness and its impact on quality of life, it is essential to consider several concepts and principles, including supercompensation, maximum recovery volume, transferability, mobility, the ten components of fitness, the seven essential movements, the three metabolic pathways, technique-consistency-intensity, and progressive overload.

Some of the Fitness Domain concepts you'll learn about are:

- **The Ten Components of Fitness:** These components include strength, endurance, power, speed, flexibility, coordination, balance, agility, accuracy, and stamina. A well-rounded fitness plan should address these components to optimize overall physical performance and health.
- **Mobility:** Mobility refers to the ability to move freely and comfortably, with resistance, through a full range of motion.

It is essential for proper exercise execution and overall physical function.

- **Seven Movements:** Squatting, lunging, hinging, pushing, pulling, carrying/walking, and twisting are fundamental human movements that should be incorporated into a fitness routine to ensure functional strength and mobility.
- **Metabolic Pathways:** Understanding the phosphagen, glycolytic, and oxidative pathways helps tailor exercise programming to target specific energy systems and improve overall conditioning.
- **Technique-Consistency-Intensity:** This progression emphasizes mastering proper technique, establishing consistent performance, and gradually increasing intensity to ensure safe and effective progress.
- **Progressive Overload:** This principle highlights the need to continuously challenge your body by gradually increasing one or more variables, such as resistance, volume, frequency, or intensity, to promote adaptation and growth.
- **Transferability:** This principle highlights the importance of selecting exercises and training modalities that positively impact your specific goals and activities.

Developing an effective fitness plan without incorporating these concepts is impossible, as they provide a comprehensive understanding of how the body responds to exercise and adapts over time. By considering these principles and tailoring workout routines accordingly, you can optimize your physical performance, reduce the risk of injury, and enhance your quality of life.

Before delving in, you must understand that your quality of life is determined by what you can do, not how much you weigh. The concepts in the Fitness Domain are built on the premise that your ability to do more things is the goal. It is the logical conclusion that if you improve what you can do, you are improving your health. This is the concept of work capacity.

Work Capacity

Work capacity is the difference between performance and function. You can do many things to improve your metabolic function that may not improve your ability to perform. Reducing insulin resistance or lowering blood pressure is great from a function perspective, but neither will help you improve your endurance, strength, or flexibility. You need to address both function and performance in the things you do to get better. This is another example of the importance of the relationship between fitness and nutrition in your journey.

Let's address the concept of work.

What is Work?

Scientifically we define work as, **W = Fd** (Work = Force x distance)

Moving an object any distance requires some application of force greater than the weight, inertia, and other variable resistances affecting that object. We have applied this principle to many aspects of our everyday life. You could say that most people define work as simply *getting things done*.

A computer programmer goes to her job every day. She sits in a chair and walks around the office. She uses her cognitive faculties to accomplish her daily tasks.

A nurse goes to the hospital and walks around for ten hours helping patients, moving people around in beds, and dealing with high-stress levels throughout his shift.

A stay-at-home mom is always on the job. She is required to be mentally quick, physically active, and able to handle a million tasks at once. She has the most demanding clientele in the world, and only the best will suffice.

Here's a secret that many people in the fitness world won't tell you. Successful FITNESS programs are NOT designed to help you lose fat, get a six-pack, or *get ripped*.

> *If you aim to get a six-pack, you aren't looking for fitness. You're looking for a six-pack.*

If the driving force behind your desire to work out is based on getting ripped, there are many places you can go and many products out there that can help you get there. Your fitness will be a secondary concern, if it's a concern at all.

Successful fitness programs focus on increasing your capacity to do work. Your body's ability to do work is directly relevant to your ability to perform at your job, in your home, and doing activities from day to day. If you are limited in how much work you can do, you hit a wall, and things go downhill. You feel tired, you can't concentrate, and you need to take longer breaks. The bottom line is less work gets done.

Basing your fitness program on increasing your ability to do work is crucial because it is the foundation for everything we do. Fitness is directly related to how much work you can do. With better fitness, that computer programmer, nurse, and stay-at-home mom can be more alert, have more energy throughout the day, handle stress, sleep better, get more done in less time, and generally feel better and be more efficient in everything they do. Fitness has nothing to do with how they look. It has everything to do with how much work they can do.

Bonus!

Guess what??? As you increase your ability to do work, you also benefit from fat loss, muscle gain, a smaller waist, and reduced clothing sizes. If you work on increasing your fitness, you will look fit. Chasing the appearance rarely achieves the same result.

Why Work Capacity is Important

Your decisions must include an evaluation of your ability to do things. Considering the impact of your choices will keep you in line with your quality of life goals and help prevent being led off track by purely aesthetic or arbitrary metrics that don't impact your long-term results. Work capacity helps with:

- **Performance Goals:** When you focus on work capacity, your health and fitness goals become about improving your performance rather than merely attaining aesthetic changes. This shift allows you to set measurable, achievable targets related to strength, endurance, flexibility, and other aspects of fitness, which can keep you motivated and consistent.

- **Enhanced Quality of Life:** Work capacity is a measure of how much you can do physically and mentally. Improving this can directly impact your daily life, making you more efficient and energetic. You'll be better equipped to handle everyday tasks, professional responsibilities, and recreational activities. This tangible impact on your daily life can motivate you to stick to your health journey.

- **Holistic Health:** By concentrating on work capacity, you consider both function (metabolic health, reducing insulin resistance, etc.) and performance (strength, endurance, etc.). This holistic approach ensures that you don't neglect important aspects of health, which can often be the case when focusing solely on weight or appearance.

- **Intrinsic Motivation:** Often, improving your work capacity leads to feeling better, having more energy, and experiencing an enhanced mood. These positive changes can provide inherent motivation, making you more likely to stay committed to your health journey in the long term.

- **Physical Changes:** As a bonus, improving your work capacity can lead to physical changes such as fat loss and muscle gain. These changes can be rewarding and motivate you to stay on track.

Remember, your health journey is not just about getting ripped or losing weight; it's about becoming fitter, stronger, and healthier overall. Focusing on work capacity ensures that you prioritize function and performance, leading to improvements in your overall quality of life.

Now, let's talk about the components of fitness.

The Ten Components of Fitness

The ten components of fitness involve a combination of physiological and neurological adaptations, as seen earlier in the Systems of Function. They must be trained through physical exertion or practiced through repetition. The first four components are physiological and need to be trained.

Physiological Adaptations (need to be trained)

- **Endurance:** This refers to the ability of the body to sustain physical activity for extended periods, regardless of the intensity or duration of the activity. It is often divided into two categories: aerobic endurance (referred to as cardiovascular fitness) and anaerobic endurance (referred to as muscular endurance). Activities that improve endurance include running, cycling, swimming, and rowing.
- **Stamina:** This refers to the ability to maintain a consistent level of physical and mental effort over time, maintaining a consistent level of intensity for as long as possible. Examples of activities that improve stamina include most interval training programs and many sports that require high levels of effort, repeated for the entire game.
- **Strength:** This refers to the force a muscle can produce in a single maximal effort. Examples of activities that improve strength include weightlifting, resistance band exercises, and bodyweight exercises such as pull-ups and chin-ups.
- **Flexibility:** This refers to the ability of the joints to move through your full range of motion. Examples of activities that improve flexibility include yoga, stretching, and activities that require a wide range of motion, such as dance and gymnastics.

The following two components are physiological and neurological and must include training and practice.

Physiological and Neurological Adaptations (need to be trained and practiced)

- **Power:** This refers to the ability to generate maximum force in a short amount of time. Power combines speed and strength. Activities that improve power include plyometric exercises such as jump squats, box jumps, sprinting, and throwing a ball.
- **Speed:** This refers to the ability to move quickly from one point to another. Speed training improves neuromuscular activation and increases fast-twitch (Type II) muscle fibers. Activities enhancing speed include sprinting, interval training, and sports like soccer and basketball.

Finally, we have the neurological components that need practice.

Neurological Adaptations (need to be practiced)

- **Coordination:** This refers to the ability to perform a series of movements smoothly and efficiently. Activities that improve coordination include dance, martial arts, and sports requiring complex movements, like tennis and volleyball.
- **Agility:** This refers to the ability to change direction quickly and effectively. Activities that improve agility include ladder drills, cone drills, and sports like basketball and soccer.
- **Balance:** This refers to maintaining equilibrium while standing or moving. Examples of activities that improve balance include yoga, tai chi, and activities that require maintaining a stable position, such as balancing on one foot or standing on a balance board.
- **Accuracy of Movement:** This refers to controlling movements precisely and accurately. Activities that improve movement accuracy include dance, gymnastics, and sports that require precise movements, such as archery and shooting.

When it comes to improving physical fitness, it's essential to work on various components to achieve a well-rounded level of fitness. Focusing solely on one aspect, such as strength training or cardio endurance, can lead to burnout and may not provide the same benefits as a more balanced approach. Here are a few reasons why working on these ten components of fitness can be beneficial:

- **More Variety Reduces Burnout:** By incorporating various activities that target different aspects of fitness, you can reduce the risk of burnout and keep your workouts interesting and engaging. For example, alternating between strength training, yoga, and running can provide a more well-rounded approach than solely focusing on one activity.

- **Increases Things to Measure and Improve:** By focusing on different components of fitness, you have more things to measure and track, which can help you set and achieve goals. For example, monitoring progress in muscular strength, endurance, and power can help you see how you're improving over time and identify areas where you may need to adjust your training.

- **Allows for More Flexibility in Managing Recovery:** Working on different components of fitness can also allow you to manage your recovery more effectively. For example, if someone is experiencing soreness or fatigue in a particular muscle group, they can shift their focus to another fitness component while that muscle group recovers. Doing so can help prevent injury and ensure that you can maintain a consistent exercise routine over time.

Focusing on these ten components of fitness can provide a more well-rounded and sustainable approach to physical fitness. By incorporating various activities and concentrating on different aspects of fitness, you can reduce the risk of burnout, track your progress, and manage your recovery more effectively.

Now, let's talk about mobility.

Mobility

Mobility is a vital component of overall physical fitness and function. Mobility is often confused with flexibility. While similar, it combines a good range of motion in the joints, flexibility in the muscles and tendons, and adequate strength to support movement, move weight, and produce or resist force in various positions. Understanding and improving mobility can help prevent injuries, enhance athletic performance, and improve the quality of daily life activities. Understanding the following is crucial to improving overall fitness:

- **Range of Motion in the Joints:** Joint range of motion refers to the full movement potential of a joint, typically its range of flexion and extension. A healthy range of motion allows for smooth and efficient movement and helps maintain joint health. For example, having a good range of motion in the hip joint enables you to perform deep squats, lunges, or step-ups with proper form and without pain or discomfort.
- **Flexibility in the Muscles and Tendons:** Flexibility refers to the ability of muscles and tendons to lengthen and stretch, allowing for a greater range of motion around a joint. Adequate flexibility helps to prevent muscle imbalances, reduces the risk of injury, and enhances overall movement quality. An example of flexibility is touching your toes, which requires lengthening of the hamstring muscles and flexibility in the lower back.
- **Adequate Strength to Support Movement:** Strength is crucial for mobility, as it allows for proper control and stability throughout the range of motion. Strength enables the body to produce and resist force, move weight, and maintain good posture during various activities. For instance, having sufficient shoulder strength allows you to maintain a proper position during a pull-up, ensuring correct technique and minimizing the risk of injury.

Consider incorporating stretching, strengthening, and balance exercises into your routine to maintain and improve mobility for daily activities. Focus on functional movements that mimic the actions performed in day-to-day tasks, such as squats, lunges, and overhead presses, to target the muscles and joints involved in these activities. When performing exercises, be sure to focus on technique and movement quality to enhance the mobility effect of each movement.

Mobility is crucial for performing daily activities with ease and comfort. Focusing on joint range of motion, muscular flexibility, and adequate strength can improve your quality of life and minimize the risk of injury during routine tasks.

The Seven Essential Movements

Our daily lives are full of constant movement. Did you know that most of these actions are variations of the same seven essential movements? By understanding and training these fundamental movements—squatting, lunging, hinging, pushing, pulling, carrying, and twisting—you can enhance your physical competence, improve your fitness level, and ensure your body is well-equipped to perform everyday tasks easily and efficiently. Let's explore these seven core movements, their relevance in your daily routines, and how integrating them into your workout program can significantly improve your quality of life.

- **Squatting** is a functional movement that is frequently used in everyday life. It's essential for maintaining lower body strength and flexibility. Daily life example: Sitting down and standing up from a chair, picking up objects from the ground, or gardening.
- **Lunging** is another functional movement important for daily activities requiring lower body strength, balance, and flexibility. Daily life example: Climbing stairs, stepping onto a curb, or picking up objects from the floor while maintaining balance.
- **Hinging (Hip Hinge)** is crucial for maintaining a strong and healthy posterior chain (back, glutes, and hamstrings), vital for functional lifting movements, and keeping a neutral spine. Daily life example: Bending down to pick up groceries, lifting a child, or reaching down to grab something from the bottom shelf.

- **Pushing movements** are commonly used in daily activities and require the strength of the chest, shoulders, and triceps. Daily life example: Opening a heavy door, pushing a shopping cart, or rearranging furniture.
- **Pulling movements** are necessary for activities that require upper body strength, specifically in the back muscles and biceps. Daily life example: Opening a drawer, pulling a wagon, or lifting a heavy object toward your body.
- **Carrying and walking** are essential activities for functional strength and endurance, as they involve moving with added weight or resistance. Daily life example: Carrying grocery bags from the store to your car, carrying a laundry basket, or carrying a child.
- **Twisting (Rotation and Anti-Rotation)** exercises involve rotation or resisting rotation of the spine and are essential for maintaining core strength and stability in daily life activities. Daily life example: Turning to look behind you while driving, lifting and twisting to put an object on a shelf, or resisting rotation when carrying an uneven load (such as a heavy bag on one shoulder).

Incorporating these seven essential movements into your exercise routine effectively improves your overall strength, flexibility, and balance, enhancing your performance in daily activities. These movements underpin many everyday tasks, from pushing open a heavy door to twisting to reach for an item on a shelf. By consciously integrating squatting, lunging, hinging, pushing, pulling, carrying, and twisting exercises into your workouts, you can ensure a well-rounded fitness routine that prepares your body for the wide variety of movements it encounters in everyday life. It's all about functional fitness – training your body to handle real-life situations as efficiently and safely as possible.

When we do various activities, we use different pathways to generate energy.

Traditional Metabolic Pathways

Our bodies are remarkable machines capable of performing a wide range of activities, from explosive bursts of power to sustained, long-term effort. This versatile functionality is primarily thanks to three distinct metabolic pathways that generate the energy necessary to fuel our muscles. From the swift and powerful phosphagen pathway, the somewhat longer-lasting glycolytic pathway, to the enduring oxidative pathway, our bodies efficiently utilize energy from different sources depending on the task at hand.

These pathways are like the gears in a car, shifting as required based on the speed and endurance needed. Let's delve into these three pathways and understand how they facilitate our everyday physical activities:

- **Super Fast Energy Pathway (Phosphagen Pathway):** This energy pathway helps us when we need to use our muscles very quickly and powerfully for a short time, like ten to fifteen seconds or less. It uses the energy stored in our muscles (ATP-CP) to help us do things like sprinting or jumping really high. An example would be running as fast as you can to catch a ball or lifting a very heavy weight, one time.

- **Fast Energy Pathway (Glycolytic Pathway):** This pathway gives us energy when doing activities that last a little longer, about ten seconds to two minutes. It uses energy from the glycogen in our body to help us do things like playing tag or doing a quick dance routine. Playing a short game of soccer with friends is a good example.

- **Slow and Steady Energy Pathway (Oxidative Pathway):** This energy pathway helps us when doing activities that last a long time, like more than two minutes. It uses energy from the fat in our body, but it needs oxygen to work. This pathway helps us during activities like jogging, swimming, or playing outside for a long time. Going for a long bike ride with your family is a great example.

These metabolic pathways—the phosphagen pathway, the glycolytic pathway, and the oxidative pathway—don't work independently in a strict on-off manner. Instead, they all function concurrently to varying degrees depending on the activity at hand.

The efficiency of your body's ability to move between each of these pathways is true Metabolic Flexibility.

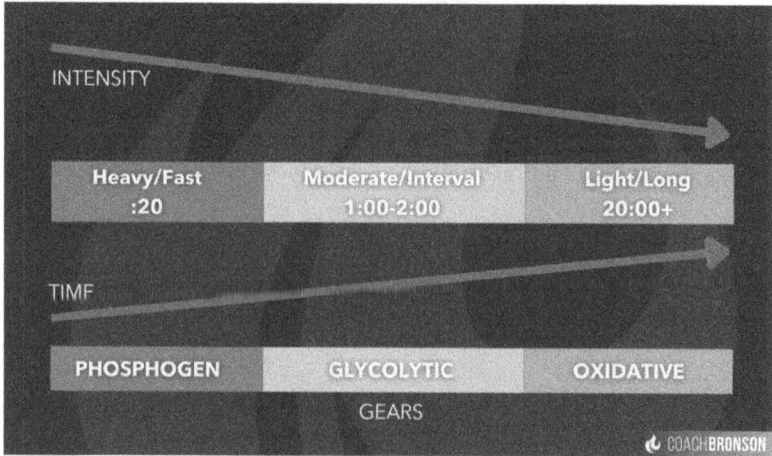

Image 11 - Metabolic pathways (as time increases, intensity decreases)

Each of these systems is always on to some degree. They overlap and complement each other. For instance, during the first few seconds of exercise, the phosphagen system is the dominant source of ATP, but the glycolytic and oxidative systems are already ramping up.

The glycolytic system becomes the primary energy provider as the phosphagen system depletes. Meanwhile, the oxidative system is gradually becoming more dominant. By the time you're several minutes into a steady-state exercise, the oxidative system is supplying the majority of the ATP.

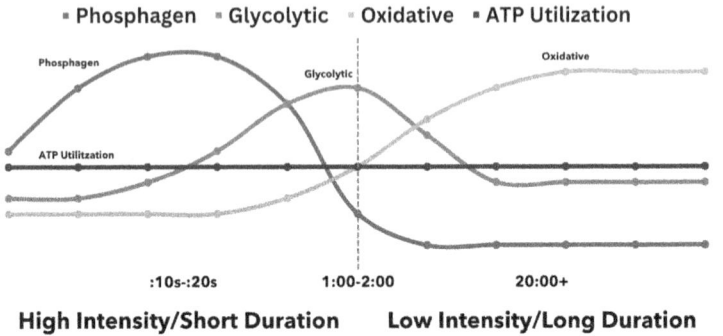

Image 12 - Metabolic Continuum

This cooperative, overlapping function of the three metabolic pathways ensures that our muscles have a continuous supply of ATP for energy, regardless of the duration or intensity of the activity. The body is a beautifully coordinated system that continually optimizes its functions to meet the current demand.

Training the Metabolic Pathways

Understanding the three metabolic pathways is an interesting part of exercise science. It helps explain how your body powers different types of physical activities. However, in practical terms, it's less important than knowing that you can improve your performance in each of these areas by simply adjusting your training.

Essentially, your body is an incredibly adaptive machine. When you consistently challenge it with varying levels of duration, speed, and resistance in your workouts, you stimulate different metabolic responses that help to improve the efficiency of these energy pathways. They are:

- **Duration:** The length of your workout or activity can dictate which energy pathway is primarily utilized. For instance, longer, low-intensity workouts improve the oxidative pathway, which uses oxygen to convert stored fat into energy. On the other hand, short, high-intensity workouts primarily stimulate the phosphagen and glycolytic pathways, improving your body's ability to perform intense bursts of activity.
- **Speed:** The faster you perform an exercise, the more you rely on the immediate energy systems (the phosphagen pathway). Training at high speeds with activities like sprinting or high-intensity interval training (HIIT) can help improve your performance in activities that require quick, explosive movements.
- **Resistance:** The more resistance you use in your workouts, the more stress you place on your muscles. This stress primarily taps into the phosphagen and glycolytic pathways. Lifting heavy weights or performing resistance exercises can help improve your strength and muscle endurance.

By manipulating these variables in your workouts, you're training your body to be more efficient across various physical tasks, from short bursts of intense effort to prolonged, steady-state exercise.

You don't necessarily need to understand the intricacies of metabolic pathways to benefit from varied exercise; you just need to challenge your body in different ways. This is a significant factor when it comes to overall metabolic conditioning and performance. The trick is to implement various techniques, consistency, and intensity.

Technique, Consistency, Intensity

When developing fitness performance, following a specific progression is essential to ensure that you build a strong foundation, avoid injuries, and improve effectively. This progression includes focusing on proper technique, consistent performance, and applying intensity. Let's break down each of these steps in a way that's easy to understand. We will start with skill and physical ability.

Skill and physical ability are two distinct but interrelated concepts in the context of sports, fitness, and physical activities. **Skill** refers to the learned ability to perform specific tasks or actions proficiently, often in a particular sport or physical activity. Skills are developed through practice, repetition, and experience, and they involve mastering certain techniques, tactics, or strategies. Skills can be both physical and mental, and they usually require a combination of cognitive understanding, body control, and fine motor skills. Examples of skills include dribbling a basketball, executing a proper swimming stroke, or performing a specific dance routine. Skills are often specific to a particular sport or activity and may not necessarily transfer directly to other sports or activities.

On the other hand, **physical ability** refers to the innate or developed physical attributes that contribute to your overall athletic performance. These attributes are often related to the health and skill-related components of fitness, such as strength, endurance, flexibility, agility, and balance. Physical abilities are more general and can be applied across various sports and activities.

Physical abilities are influenced by factors such as genetics, training, nutrition, and overall health. By improving physical abilities, you can enhance your performance across a range of sports and activities. For example, increasing muscular strength can benefit an individual in activities like weightlifting, sprinting, and even swimming.

In summary, skill refers to the learned ability to perform specific tasks proficiently, often involving the mastery of techniques, tactics, or strategies. In contrast, physical ability refers to the innate or developed physical attributes contributing to overall athletic performance. Both skill and physical ability are essential for success in sports and physical activities, and they often work together to help you reach your full potential. Developing both skill and physical ability through practice, training, and proper guidance can lead to improved performance and a more enjoyable experience in sports and fitness. This is where technique, consistency, and intensity enter the picture. Let's start with technique.

Proper Technique

The first step in improving your fitness performance is to learn and practice the correct technique for each exercise. This means understanding how to perform each movement safely and effectively, using the correct posture and form. Practicing proper technique helps prevent injuries and ensures that you target the right muscles during each exercise. For example, if you are learning to do a squat, keeping your chest up, your back straight, and your knees tracking over your toes as you lower your body is essential.

Focusing on technique is crucial for enhancing the neurological components of fitness, such as balance, coordination, accuracy of movement, speed, and agility. By practicing proper form and movement patterns, you train your brain and nervous system to communicate effectively with your muscles, improving performance. Here's how a focus on technique impacts these neurological components of fitness.

Consistent Performance

Once you have mastered the proper technique for each exercise, the next step is to focus on consistent performance. This means regularly practicing the exercises and maintaining good form throughout each workout. Consistency helps build muscle memory, making it easier to perform the exercises correctly each time.

To develop consistent performance, create a workout routine that includes each of the exercises you've learned and practice them regularly. As you become more comfortable with the movements, you can gradually increase the repetitions or sets you perform during each workout.

Consistent performance of proper technique is essential for enhancing the physiological components of fitness, such as strength, stamina, endurance, flexibility, and power. You can effectively target the right muscles and systems by practicing and maintaining correct form and movement patterns, improving overall fitness.

Proper technique and consistent performance are crucial, but intensity is often the missing link.

Applying Intensity

There are three things to consider when talking about intensity:

- **Absolute Intensity** is the work you are doing. If you move 100 pounds, then you just moved 100 pounds. If you ran one mile, then you just ran one mile. That's it. The measurable work completed is the absolute intensity.

- **Relative Intensity** is the percentage of the effort required to complete the work based on your fitness level. If the most you can move is 200 pounds and you move 100 pounds, your relative intensity is fifty percent. If Nancy can move 400 pounds and she moves 100 pounds, then her relative intensity is twenty-five percent. Any fitness program should focus on increasing your ability in both Absolute and Relative Intensity.

- **The Rate of Perceived Exertion (RPE)** is the one that gets people all messed up, and this is where we're going to focus our discussion. RPE is 100 percent based on how hard you FEEL you are working. When most people talk about intensity in a workout, they talk about RPE. They say, "That workout crushed me!" It's a subjective observation about how much energy they feel they put into the work. It's the same when someone says, "Oh, that wasn't so bad; I could do more." These two points of view can and often do exist simultaneously. They're related.

When you first start a new fitness routine, everything seems hard. You aren't worried about how much weight you're using or how fast you do the work. You're just concerned with getting through the workout. You want to perform the movements safely and correctly. That's where your focus is and should be.

When your Absolute and Relative Intensities are low and your RPE is high, everything seems hard. After a while, you get more comfortable with the movements and sense that you can go faster or use a heavier weight. Your Absolute and Relative Intensities are increasing. As these increase, your RPE decreases. The work feels easier even though you may be doing more measurable work. The key is to find a way to increase your RPE again. Increasing the level of effort is the key to improving your overall fitness.

Here's the kicker—

How do you know when this happens and what to do about it? If the work feels easier, you should make it more challenging, right? Isn't that what getting better is all about?

As you get more in shape, the amount of work you can do should increase. How hard it feels to do that work should stay the same. I can't count how often I've heard a relatively new person tell me that the workouts aren't challenging.

"I'm getting bored. The workouts aren't hard enough."

My response was, "Then make it harder."

What's written in the program does not determine how hard you work or the effort you put into it. If you feel like the workouts are easy, it's because you're getting better!

Now, go make it hard again!

If your fitness program is working, you will and should reach a period where things seem easier than they did before. You will know this by how you feel. If you are tracking your performance, you'll know it by looking at the evidence in the numbers. If you aren't tracking your performance, knowing when to increase your RPE through additional Relative Intensity in your workouts will be tough. You won't know how fast you did this workout last time, so you can try and go faster this time. You won't know what weight you used last time, so that you can use a heavier weight this time. Anyone not tracking their performance is not serious about improving their health. It's the most critical part of the process.

Before moving on, I have one more point about intensity. It is that you can and will get better by focusing on three things.

Getting Better in Three Parts

Three things affect or create intensity that you can use to improve your fitness and get more out of your workouts. They are:

- **Technique:** Focus on getting better at executing a movement. The better you perform a movement, the more you'll get out of it.
- **Resistance:** Lifting or moving more weight than before is a hallmark for improving your fitness. How can you expect gains if you always pick up the same dumbbell?
- **Time:** The speed at which you move is a sure-fire way to get more intensity into your workouts. How much more speed? Only your past performance can tell you that.

Past performance is the map that will guide you to improved health and fitness.

The Technique, Resistance, or Time

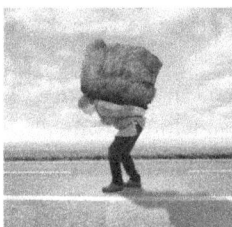

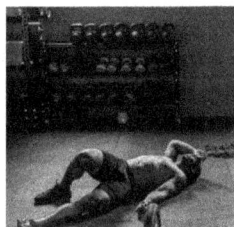

Applied to you   You apply   Feel you apply

Image 13 - Applied Intensity

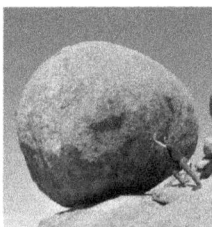

Here's the cool part of the whole process. Intensity works two ways! You can increase it or decrease it as needed. Because fitness is a personal journey, each person has different needs. While one person may seek more intensity, another may need less. Someone new to fitness needs less intensity as your body and central nervous system grow into the new routine. A person who just had back surgery needs a level of intensity that their newly repaired body can handle without breaking again. A competitive athlete will likely look for more intensity in their program.

After establishing proper technique and consistent performance, it's time to apply intensity to your workouts. You can increase intensity in various ways, such as adding more weight, increasing the number of repetitions or sets, or reducing the rest time between sets. By increasing the intensity of your workouts, you will challenge your muscles and cardiovascular system, leading to improvements in strength, endurance, and overall fitness.

It's important to remember that increasing intensity should be done gradually and safely. Always listen to your body and avoid pushing yourself too hard, too quickly. This will help prevent injuries and ensure you continue progressing in your fitness journey.

Following the progression of proper technique, consistent performance, and applying intensity allows for safe and effective increases in the stimuli applied to the body. This approach ensures that the foundation is built before increasing the challenge, minimizing the risk of injury, and optimizing the benefits of exercise. This progression ties directly into progressive overload and improving physical performance.

The progression of developing fitness performance involves first learning and practicing proper technique, then focusing on consistent performance, and finally applying intensity to your workouts. By following this progression, you will build a strong foundation for your fitness journey, minimize the risk of injuries, and maximize your potential for improvement. But remember, everyone starts at a different place.

Beginners vs. Veterans

A beginner in the world of fitness has more work to do in developing their neurological system compared to someone who has already established the skills needed to apply greater stimuli to the physiological system. The primary focus for beginners is learning and mastering proper technique, which is crucial for developing the neurological components of fitness, such as balance, coordination, accuracy of movement, and agility. There are three stages of progression: beginner, transition, and advanced.

Beginner Stage

This stage focuses on developing the neurological system. For beginners, the initial phase of their fitness journey is primarily focused on developing the neurological system to enable better physiological adaptation. This involves learning and practicing the proper technique for various exercises, which helps establish the neuromuscular connections necessary for effective and safe movements.

At this stage, beginners will see more skill-based results as their bodies adapt to new movements and activities. During this phase, beginners often experience rapid improvements in skill acquisition, coordination, and balance as their nervous system adapts to the new stimulus. As they become more proficient in executing exercises with correct form, the risk of injury is minimized, and they lay a solid foundation for future progress. Once the neurological system is developed, a beginner will move to the second stage.

Transition Stage

This stage is about shifting focus to physiological adaptations. As beginners progress and become more proficient in the skills needed for various exercises, their focus will gradually shift to managing physiological stimuli. At this stage, their nervous system has adapted to the new demands, and they can now safely apply greater stimulus to the physiological system. This involves increasing intensity, volume, frequency, or other variables to promote progressive overload.

Progressive Overload - The 1% Rule

Progressive overload is a fundamental principle in fitness that states in order to improve physical performance, the body must be subjected to a stimulus greater than what it is accustomed to. This concept encourages gradual increases in one or more variables, such as resistance, volume, frequency, or intensity, to challenge the body to adapt and grow stronger.

Safely implementing progressive overload is crucial for ensuring consistent progress and minimizing the risk of injury.

From a beginner's standpoint, the idea of progressive overload might seem daunting, but it's essential to understand that it doesn't necessarily require a significant increase in stimulus. This is where **the 1% Rule** comes into play. **The 1% Rule** suggests that improving physical ability doesn't require much effort; instead, it just takes a little more than what is already being done. By focusing on small, incremental improvements, beginners can safely and effectively progress in their fitness journey.

Here are some ways to implement progressive overload safely, particularly for beginners:

- **Focus on Proper Technique:** Before increasing the stimulus, it is vital to master proper technique for each exercise. This ensures that you target the right muscles, optimize energy usage, and minimize the risk of injury. By first focusing on technique, you create a solid foundation upon which you can safely and effectively build.

- **Gradual Increases:** As a beginner, it's crucial to avoid making large jumps in intensity, volume, or resistance. Instead, apply **the 1% Rule** and focus on making small, manageable increases in the variables. For example, you might add one more rep to your workout, increase the weight you're lifting by a small increment, or shorten rest periods slightly.

- **Listen to Your Body:** Always pay attention to how your body feels and responds to the increased stimulus. If you experience pain, excessive fatigue, or signs of overtraining, scale back the intensity and give your body time to recover. Remember, consistent progress is better than pushing too hard and risking injury or burnout.

- **Mix It Up:** While the focus should be on gradually increasing the stimulus, it's also essential to vary your workouts to prevent boredom and keep your body challenged. Incorporate different exercises, training modalities, and workout structures to maintain your motivation and ensure well-rounded fitness development.

- **Be Patient and Consistent:** Progress takes time, and it's essential to be patient with yourself as you implement progressive overload. Consistency is key – stick to your workout routine and trust that the small, incremental improvements will add up over time, leading to noticeable gains in strength, endurance, and overall fitness.

Progressive overload is a fundamental principle in fitness that encourages gradual increases in the stimuli applied to the body to promote adaptation and growth. For beginners, **the 1% Rule** demonstrates that improving physical ability doesn't require much effort, just a little more than what is already being done. By focusing on proper technique, gradual increases, and listening to your body, you can safely and effectively implement progressive overload, leading to consistent progress in your fitness journey.

The results of your fitness activities will become more physically apparent as your body adapts to the increased demands by improving strength, endurance, flexibility, and power. Beginners will spend more time working on the physiological aspects of fitness, fine-tuning their workouts to optimize physical adaptations. From there, they will progress to the advanced stage.

Advanced Stage

This stage is about balancing skill maintenance and physiological progress. As you progress in your fitness journey, you must maintain the skills you have developed while continuing to challenge your physiological systems. This involves regularly incorporating skill-based exercises to keep your neurological system sharp and adapting your workouts to ensure progressive overload and continuous improvement in your physical performance.

Beginners in fitness will initially focus on developing their neurological system through skill acquisition, spending more time learning and practicing proper technique. As they progress, the emphasis will shift to managing physiological stimuli, resulting in more visible physical results.

By following this progression, you can safely and effectively improve your fitness levels, enhance your overall well-being, and reduce the risk of injury.

Scaling

Scaling and modifications play a crucial role in tailoring workouts to suit a person's individual needs and abilities, allowing for an adequate adaptation without exceeding your capacity. By adjusting the intensity, complexity, resistance, speed, or reps, scaling and modifications can cater to both physiological and neurological stimulus requirements, ensuring optimal progress and minimizing the risk of injury or burnout. Let's explore how you can apply these adjustments to increase and decrease intensity based on your needs.

Here are some key points highlighting the importance of scaling and modifications in a fitness plan:

- **Accessibility:** Fitness plans should be accessible to individuals of different fitness levels, ages, and abilities. Scaling exercises make them more achievable for beginners or those with physical limitations. It allows individuals to start at a comfortable level and gradually progress as their strength, endurance, and skills improve.
- **Injury Prevention:** Scaling and modifications help reduce the risk of injuries during exercise. Adapting exercises to an individual's current capabilities ensures that movements are performed with proper form and within a safe range of motion. It allows individuals to work within their physical limitations while still challenging themselves appropriately.
- **Progression:** Scaling and modifications enable gradual progression in a fitness plan. As individuals become stronger and more proficient, they can increase exercise intensity, complexity, or resistance. This progressive approach promotes continued improvements in strength, endurance, and overall fitness.

- **Individual Goals:** Fitness plans should align with an individual's specific goals. Scaling and modifications allow for customization based on personal objectives. Whether the aim is to build strength, increase flexibility, lose weight, or improve cardiovascular fitness, scaling exercises ensures that the workout plan aligns with the desired outcomes.
- **Variability and Adaptability:** Fitness plans should be adaptable to changing circumstances and individual needs. Scaling exercises provide the flexibility to modify workouts based on time constraints, available equipment, or physical conditions. It allows for versatility in designing workouts that suit different situations without compromising progress or effectiveness.
- **Continual Challenge:** Scaling and modifications ensure that workouts remain challenging and engaging over time. By adjusting variables such as resistance, repetitions, or range of motion, individuals can continue to push their limits, avoid plateaus, and stimulate further improvements. It promotes a sense of accomplishment and motivation to keep progressing.

When scaling exercises to make them more attainable, individuals can focus on reducing intensity, decreasing weights or resistance, shortening the duration, or modifying the range of motion. This approach allows beginners or those recovering from injuries to safely participate in workouts and gradually build strength and endurance.

On the other hand, scaling to increase intensity or complexity involves adding resistance, progressing to more challenging variations, expanding the range of motion, or incorporating advanced techniques. This ensures that workouts remain stimulating for individuals who have already developed a certain fitness and skill level.

Overall, scaling and modifications are essential tools in following a fitness plan. They enable customization, reduce the risk of injury, support gradual progression, and ensure that workouts align with individual goals and abilities. By incorporating scaling techniques, individuals can create a sustainable and effective fitness plan that evolves with their needs and promotes long-term success.

Scaling and modifications are done through three primary means. They are:

- **Decreasing Intensity:** For beginners or those recovering from injury, it may be necessary to decrease the intensity of exercises to ensure safe and effective progress. Scaling and modifications can involve simplifying complex movements, reducing the resistance (weight or load), slowing down the speed of execution, or decreasing the number of reps performed. For example, a beginner may start with bodyweight squats instead of weighted squats or perform push-ups with knees on the ground instead of a full push-up. These modifications allow the person to work on your technique and build strength while avoiding excessive stress on your body.

- **Increasing Intensity:** As you progress in your fitness journey and become more proficient in executing exercises with proper technique, scaling and modifications can be applied to increase the intensity of workouts. This can involve adding complexity to movements, increasing resistance, speeding up the execution, or increasing the number of reps or sets performed. For example, an advanced exerciser might progress from regular push-ups to decline push-ups, or incorporate plyometric elements like jump squats. These adjustments challenge the body to adapt and grow stronger, improving both the physiological and neurological aspects of fitness.

- **Balancing Physiological and Neurological Stimuli:** Scaling and modifications allow for individual application of physiological and neurological stimuli, ensuring that exercises are tailored to the person's current fitness level and goals. By adjusting the intensity, complexity, resistance, speed, or reps, you can focus on the aspects of fitness that require the most attention, whether improving technique, balance, and coordination (neurological stimulus) or building strength, endurance, and power (physiological stimulus).

Scaling and modifications are essential tools for creating individualized workouts that cater to a person's specific needs and abilities. By adjusting intensity, complexity, resistance, speed, or reps, these adaptations allow for adequate progression without exceeding the individual's capacity, ensuring a safe and effective fitness journey. These adjustments can be applied to increase and decrease intensity based on the person's current fitness level, goals, and limitations, allowing for a tailored approach to achieving optimal health and well-being.

Now, if you didn't get the subtle hint, scaling and modifications are not only beneficial but necessary. Both are crucial when it comes to transferability. All work in harmony for overall and sustainable well-being and health. But what do we mean by transferability?

Transferability

Transferability is a cousin of technique. It's the concept that certain training principles, movement patterns, or exercises can positively impact other aspects of training, even if they are not directly related. The idea that "everything we train, trains everything we train," means that the skills and movement patterns developed in one exercise or activity can be beneficial and translate to other exercises or activities.

The movement pattern is often more beneficial to learn than the exercise itself because mastering a fundamental movement pattern can be applied to various exercises and activities. This transferability reinforces skill development and saves time by increasing the reps without increasing the work.

For example, take the double overhand grip versus the mixed grip on barbell work. The double overhand grip can have greater transferability to other exercises because it promotes symmetry and balance in the body. This movement strengthens grip and forearm muscles, which can be beneficial in various activities such as pull-ups, deadlifts, and rows. In contrast, the mixed grip might provide a firmer grip for specific exercises like heavy deadlifts. Still, it may not offer the same level of transferability as other exercises due to its asymmetrical nature.

Another example is the hip hinge movement pattern, used in several exercises such as deadlifts, kettlebell swings, and Romanian deadlifts. By learning and perfecting the hip hinge, you develop a strong foundation that can be transferred to various exercises, improving your overall training efficiency. Mastering the hip hinge can also help prevent injuries by ensuring proper form and engagement of the correct muscle groups.

Transferability is valuable because it allows you to:

- **Reinforce Skill Development**: As you learn and practice fundamental movement patterns, you develop skills that can be applied to various exercises, activities, and sports, improving performance and versatility.
- **Save Time and Effort:** By focusing on transferable movement patterns, you can make your training more efficient, maximizing the benefits without necessarily increasing the workload.
- **Prevent Injuries:** Understanding and applying transferable movement patterns ensures you use proper form and engage the right muscle groups during exercises, reducing the risk of injury.
- **Enhance Overall Fitness:** Transferable movement patterns and exercises help improve overall fitness by targeting multiple muscle groups and aspects of physical performance.

The concept of transferability highlights the importance of learning and mastering fundamental movement patterns rather than focusing solely on specific exercises. This approach reinforces skill development, saves time and effort, prevents injuries, and enhances overall fitness, making training more efficient and effective. But what about nutrition, how does that interact with fitness to improve health?

Let's dig into that.

Takeaways

- Your fitness is determined by what you can do not how you look.
- Understanding fitness exponentially increases your measures of success

- Technique and consistency will do more for you than Intensity. You still need intensity to push you forward.
- It's easier to see progress as a beginner. If that's your excuse for not getting started, you've got it backwards.

Resources

- Get **FREE** Bonus material that includes a complete breakdown and analysis of the most common fitness and nutrition programs to help you evaluate which ones will work best for you by following the F2 Method.
- Join **Coach Bronson's Body Confident Support Group** on Discord and meet more people who are improving themselves every day. https://discord.coachbronson.com
- Download the **FREE Body Confident Book Bonus Material** and Community information at https://bodyconfidentbook.com.

CHAPTER 9

NUTRITION DOMAIN CONCEPTS AND PRINCIPLES

"It's all about nutrition. You can train, train, train all you want, but I always say you can't out-train a bad diet." ~ Joe Wicks

Nutrition is a fundamental aspect of overall well-being, influencing physical vitality, mental clarity, and disease prevention. It is the foundation for optimal health, allowing us to achieve peak performance, maintain an efficient metabolism, and promote general wellness. Exploring various concepts and principles is crucial to unlock the power of nutrition and its impact on our bodies. This section will delve into key nutrition concepts, including inflammation, metabolic rate, fat adaptation, electrolytes, hydration, thresholds vs. ratios, metabolic flexibility, macros, meal frequency and timing, and the purpose of fat and protein.

Let's take a closer look at these nutrition domain concepts:

- **Inflammation:** Is it Good or Bad? This concept explores the complex nature of inflammation in our bodies and how it can both support and hinder our well-being. We will examine the role of nutrition in managing inflammation and promoting a balanced immune response.
- **Metabolic Rate:** In this intriguing concept, we challenge the common notion of a fixed metabolic rate and uncover the

dynamic nature of our metabolism. We'll explore how nutrition influences our metabolic processes and debunk misconceptions surrounding this topic.

- **Fat Adaptation:** Discover the transformative power of fat adaptation as we delve into using fat as a primary fuel source. We'll explore the benefits, considerations, and strategies for optimizing fat adaptation through nutrition.
- **Hydration:** Learn about the vital role of electrolytes and proper hydration in maintaining optimal health and performance. We'll explore the importance of electrolyte balance, hydration strategies, and how nutrition significantly supports hydration needs.
- **Thresholds vs. Ratios:** This concept examines the delicate balance between macronutrient thresholds and ratios for optimal performance. We'll explore how understanding and manipulating these thresholds affect our body composition, energy levels, and overall well-being.
- **Metabolic Flexibility:** Unlock metabolic flexibility, efficiently switching between different fuel sources. We'll explore nutrition strategies that enhance metabolic flexibility and promote adaptability in the face of changing dietary and lifestyle demands.
- **Macros Are Not Nutrition**: Challenge the belief that macronutrients alone define nutrition. We'll dive deeper into the importance of micronutrients and other essential elements that contribute to a well-rounded and nourishing diet.
- **Meal Frequency and Timing:** Explore the concept of meal frequency and timing, including popular approaches such as fasting, one meal a day (OMAD), and two meals a day (2MAD). We'll delve into the potential benefits and considerations of these approaches and how you can integrate them into a personalized nutrition plan.
- **Fat and Protein:** In this concept, we'll dissect the roles of fat and protein in our diets and their distinct purposes within our bodies. We'll explore the importance of quality sources, proper amounts, and their impact on our overall health and performance.

By understanding and applying these nutrition concepts and principles, we can optimize our dietary choices, support our body's natural functions, and unlock our full potential for vibrant health and peak performance. Join us on this enlightening journey as we delve into the intricate world of nutrition and its transformative power.

Inflammation, Good or Bad?

Inflammation is a vital part of the body's immune response, a defense mechanism the body employs when it experiences an injury or infection. Think of it like your body's internal fire department.

When there's a problem, such as a tissue injury or infection, cells in your body send out an alarm, like a 911 call. Immune cells, including white blood cells, are the firefighters. They rush to the scene to limit damage, clear away the debris, and start the repair process. The signs of this response are the redness, heat, swelling, and pain you experience at an injury or infection site. This is akin to seeing fire trucks, firefighters, and hoses at work at the scene of a fire, trying to control and extinguish it.

Inflammation is beneficial and necessary because injuries wouldn't heal without it, and minor infections could become life-threatening. Much like how we rely on firefighters to put out fires, we rely on the inflammation process to address injuries and infections in our bodies.

However, problems arise when inflammation goes on for too long or happens when it's not needed. This is like a fire department constantly called out to the same fire, or even worse, false alarms. The firefighters get tired, resources are wasted, and they can't attend to other fires that might need their attention.

In terms of the body, this extended inflammation, known as chronic inflammation, can start to damage healthy cells, tissues, and organs over time. It's essentially the body's immune system attacking its own cells because it's constantly in firefighting mode. This can lead to various health issues like heart disease, diabetes, arthritis, and even cancer.

Unhealthy or chronic inflammation symptoms can be persistent fatigue, constant low-grade fever, body pain, skin rashes, or abdominal pain. These can be likened to a city constantly covered in smoke, even when there are no fires because the firefighting operations have become misguided and overzealous.

Inflammation, like a fire department, is a necessary and beneficial part of our defense mechanism; it is crucial that it operates accurately. Too much of it, or at the wrong time, can lead to significant health problems, just as a fire department constantly responding to false alarms or being unable to extinguish fires effectively would cause damage to the city it's supposed to protect.

The food choices you make can significantly impact the level of inflammation in your body. In essence, a diet rich in nutrient-dense, bioavailable, and satiating foods like meat and eggs and low in processed foods and industrial seed oils can help reduce unnecessary inflammation.

- **Nutrient-Dense Foods**: Foods like meat and eggs are high in various nutrients that your body needs to function optimally. They contain essential amino acids, minerals, and vitamins, many of which have anti-inflammatory effects. For instance, omega-3 fatty acids, found in certain types of fish, have strong anti-inflammatory properties.
- **Bioavailability:** Bioavailability refers to the proportion of a nutrient absorbed from the diet and used for normal body functions. Animal proteins like meat and eggs are highly bioavailable, meaning your body can efficiently use their nutrients. In comparison, some plant-based protein sources may have lower bioavailability, meaning your body has to work hard to benefit from them. More work means more stress and inflammation.
- **Satiating Foods:** Foods high in protein, like meat and eggs, are incredibly satiating. The hormone response to these foods is balanced and is less likely to cause extra stress on your system from poor hormone signaling.
- **Avoiding Processed Foods:** Processed foods often contain additives, preservatives, and other chemicals that can trigger an inflammatory response in the body. They are also generally high

in unhealthy fats and sugars, which are linked to inflammation when consumed in excess.

- **Cutting Out Industrial Seed Oils:** Industrial seed oils, such as soybean, corn, and sunflower oils, are toxic, rancid, high in trans fat, and oxidize very easily. They are also high in linoleic acids. While linoleic acids are essential, they can promote inflammation when consumed in excess, especially when the balance with omega-3 fatty acids (found in fish, meat, and eggs) is skewed.

By focusing on nutrient-dense, bioavailable, and satiating foods, and cutting out processed foods and industrial seed oils, you maintain a well-balanced diet that can help regulate your body's inflammatory response. It's akin to providing the right resources and efficient management to your 'internal fire department,' enabling it to respond to and resolve 'fire incidents' effectively without causing unnecessary damage.

Metabolic Rate is a Red Herring

When people speak about metabolism, they are referring to metabolic rate, typically measured as the number of calories your body burns at rest (basal metabolic rate or BMR). However, metabolism involves a broad range of chemical processes in the body, and the metabolic rate, or BMR, only represents a portion of this.

Traditionally, the metabolic rate measures the speed at which our body burns calories. A fast metabolism is often associated with thinness, and a slow metabolism with obesity. However, this is an oversimplification and doesn't account for the complexity of metabolic processes and how they impact overall health and body composition.

The human body uses energy (from the food we eat) not only for physical activity but also for a multitude of biochemical reactions necessary for life. These include synthesizing new molecules, recycling old ones, maintaining the electric potential of nerve cells, maintaining body temperature, and various other processes.

While a higher metabolic rate can potentially aid weight loss (because you're using material more quickly), it doesn't necessarily equate to better health or optimal metabolic performance. In fact, some studies suggest that a higher metabolic rate may be linked with an increased rate of aging and a shorter lifespan.

A more complete understanding of metabolic health encompasses not just the speed of energy consumption but also the efficiency of various physiological systems and biochemical reactions in the body. A more efficient metabolism can use less energy to accomplish the same tasks, whereas an inefficient metabolism uses more energy.

Trying to increase your metabolic rate is similar to REDUCING your gas mileage. That doesn't really make sense, does it?

The nutrients we consume not only provide energy but also supply the body with the raw materials necessary for all these various metabolic processes. For example, proteins provide amino acids for tissue repair, thyroid hormones, and the building of enzymes. Fats are essential for hormone production and cell membrane integrity. Vitamins and minerals are crucial cofactors in countless biochemical reactions.

Various factors, including genetics, physical activity levels, diet, stress, sleep, and more influence the complexity and efficiency of metabolic processes. A better approach to improving metabolic health would be to focus on optimizing these factors rather than solely focusing on the speed at which the body uses up the food we eat.

If you were a car

Looking at metabolic rate in terms of calories burned is akin to measuring a car's performance by its miles per gallon. It doesn't tell you how fast the car is, how well it handles in the corners, or if the brakes are working as required.

Many components must work together harmoniously for a car to run efficiently and reliably. The engine, transmission, brakes, tires, electrical system, cooling system, and more all play a vital role. Similarly, in the body, different systems, like the cardiovascular, nervous, endocrine, and digestive systems, contribute to overall metabolic health.

Just as a car needs more than gasoline to function optimally (oil, coolant, brake fluid, etc.), the body needs more than energy. It requires a variety of nutrients (proteins, fats, vitamins, and minerals) to support the myriad of biochemical reactions happening in the body. Oil doesn't provide fuel for the vehicle to move, but it's essential for the engine's health and efficiency. It reduces friction and wear, helps disperse heat, and keeps the engine clean. In our body, things like vitamins and minerals are similar. They don't provide energy themselves, but they act as cofactors in enzymatic reactions, supporting the 'engine' of our cells and helping maintain our health.

Brake pads and rotors are like our body's ability to control inflammation. We need some inflammation for healing, just like a car needs brakes to slow down. But if the inflammation gets out of control or the brakes are constantly rubbing, it can lead to problems.

Transmission fluid could be compared to hormones in our body. Just like the fluid helps shift gears and keep the car running smoothly, hormones help regulate different bodily functions and keep everything in balance.

Spark plugs could be likened to neurons in our nervous system, igniting the 'spark' that sends signals throughout the body, just as a spark plug ignites the fuel in a car.

In the same way that a mechanic wouldn't only consider miles per gallon when evaluating a car's overall performance, we shouldn't only consider metabolic rate when evaluating metabolic health. Just as a well-maintained vehicle performs better, a body supported by regular exercise, a nutrient-dense diet, and a healthy lifestyle will have a healthier and more efficient metabolism.

The concept of metabolic rate is not flawed per se, but it's just one part of the much larger, more complex picture of metabolic health. Metabolic rate plays a role in energy balance and body composition, but the concept is limited. A more holistic understanding of metabolism considers the variety of processes at play and their efficiency. Nutrition should be recognized as providing the building blocks for these processes, not just fuel.

Thresholds vs. Fixed Ratios

While conventional wisdom dictates specific ratios of macronutrients, an individual's needs can deviate substantially from these standards. Adhering to fixed ratios could result in fat or protein being too high or too low based on individual needs, leading to nutrient imbalance and health issues.

Revisit the car example. You need both oil and gasoline for your car to run efficiently. If you consider gasoline like dietary fat and oil like dietary protein, both are necessary for the vehicle (your body) to run properly.

However, maintaining a specific ratio of oil to gasoline doesn't make sense for the car's functionality. For example, it doesn't work to say you need a particular percentage of oil to gas, such as a thirty:seventy ratio. Too much oil (protein) might overpressure the engine, while too much gasoline (fat) might flood it. Both situations could result in the car malfunctioning or even breaking down.

Instead, your car requires specific amounts of both oil and gasoline. The oil keeps the engine parts lubricated and functioning smoothly, while gasoline fuels the car's movement. These amounts aren't relational, as they serve different roles and have different usage rates.

Similarly, we can't rely on fixed ratios of fat to protein in nutrition. Individuals might need more or less of either nutrient based on their unique physiology, activity levels, and metabolic health. Using a set ratio can lead to an overabundance or shortage of either nutrient.

Manage macros independently of each other

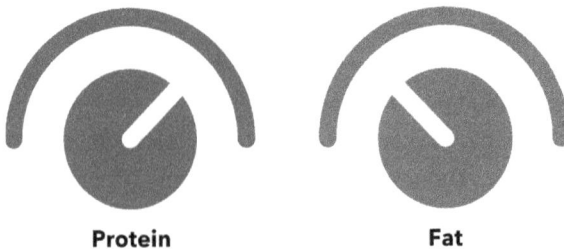

Protein   **Fat**

Figure 15 - Macros are Individual Requirements

Instead of adhering to rigid ratios, we should determine individual thresholds or specific needs for both fat and protein, much like the individual needs for oil and gasoline in a car. This way, we can tailor our diets to meet our unique nutritional needs, promoting optimal health and well-being.

Personalized nutrition, considering individual thresholds for fat and protein, appears to be a more beneficial approach. Due to their unique metabolic makeup, some people might require more protein or fat to maintain muscle mass or control blood sugar levels, while others might need less.

Neurological Implications

Fats, particularly omega-3 fatty acids, have profound effects on brain health. They are essential for brain function, memory, and cognitive skills and help fight mental disorders such as depression and anxiety. Proteins, on the other hand, are crucial for neurotransmitter synthesis. For instance, tryptophan, an amino acid, is the precursor for serotonin, the feel-good neurotransmitter.

Biological and Physiological Functions

Fats play a significant role in maintaining cell membrane integrity, synthesizing hormones, and providing an efficient energy source. Protein is equally critical and involved in nearly every cellular function. It gives structure to cells, plays a vital role in immune function, and is instrumental in muscle growth and repair.

A nutrition plan that respects individual differences will likely succeed in the long run. By moving away from the one-size-fits-all ratio approach, we can develop a more nuanced understanding of our nutritional needs, focusing not only on macronutrients but also on the richness and diversity of micronutrients that truly constitute a balanced diet.

While macros, particularly fats and proteins, are vital to our dietary needs, they alone do not define nutrition. Balancing these with a rich array of micronutrients for overall health is crucial. A shift towards individualized nutrient needs, rather than fixed ratios, can allow for a more effective, personalized, and nutrient-dense approach to eating.

Macros Are Not Nutrition

In the realm of dietary principles, macronutrients—notably proteins, fats, and carbohydrates—often reign supreme. Of course, macronutrients are undeniably crucial for our health. Proteins are the building blocks for muscle growth, enzymes, hormones, and recovery. Fats are vital for hormone production, cell structure, energy transportation, and the absorption of fat-soluble vitamins. However, merely focusing on the quantity of these macros can often overshadow the quality and diversity of nutrients we consume.

Many dietary programs and guidelines center their strategies around manipulating these macros to achieve various fitness and health goals. While these macronutrients are essential in body composition and metabolic performance, focusing solely on macros can distort our perspective of accurate nutrition.

Even though fat and protein macros are important, nutrient density should be the primary consideration for a healthy diet. Our bodies require a spectrum of vitamins, minerals, antioxidants, and other micronutrients for optimal function. Focusing on macros alone may lead to a diet lacking these critical micronutrients, leading to potential deficiencies and poor health outcomes.

For example, chicken breast has a fantastic lean protein-to-fat ratio to help with body composition. However, it's horribly lacking in most nutrients and is high in Omega 6 fats. Neither makes it a good choice as a staple of good nutrition.

The key to proper nutrition and better health outcomes isn't solely about macros but also about incorporating diverse nutrient-dense foods into our diets. Doing so can prevent deficiencies, promote overall health, and optimize body composition more effectively.

Measuring Nutrition

Measuring nutrition extends far beyond merely tracking the nutrients we consume. It involves a comprehensive understanding of our body's ability to digest, absorb, and utilize these nutrients effectively, as well as the consequent effects on our health and well-being. This holistic approach to nutrition evaluation accounts for individual variations in metabolism, genetic factors, gut health, and lifestyle.

Nutrient absorption is a critical factor in measuring nutrition. Even with a nutrient-rich diet, if your body isn't effectively digesting and absorbing those nutrients, your health won't benefit. Factors like gut health, the presence of certain enzymes, and even stress levels can influence nutrient absorption. For instance, insufficient stomach acid can impair protein digestion, and certain gut disorders like celiac disease can inhibit the absorption of numerous nutrients.

It's also crucial to consider the bioavailability of nutrients, which refers to the proportion of a nutrient absorbed and utilized in the body. Not all nutrients are equally bioavailable due to interactions with other compounds, the presence of enhancers or inhibitors, and an individual's nutritional status. For example, the iron in plant-based foods is less bioavailable than iron from animal sources.

Measuring nutrition also involves observing the effects on your health. This could include changes in energy levels, body composition, skin health, mood, cognitive function, and even lab results like blood glucose levels or lipid profiles. Tracking these changes can provide valuable insights into whether your diet meets your unique nutritional needs and promotes optimal health.

Tracking your nutrient intake, evaluating your body's ability to absorb and utilize those nutrients, and understanding their impacts on your health may seem complex, but here are some practical examples of how you can do this:

- **Track Nutrient Intake:** This is often the first step. Use a food diary or a nutrition tracking app to record everything you eat and drink. These tools can help you see your macronutrient intake and the variety of vitamins and minerals in your diet. Try to include a variety of foods in your diet to cover all essential nutrients.

- **Improve Digestion and Absorption:** Chew your food thoroughly to aid digestion. Including probiotic foods like yogurt, kefir, sauerkraut, and kimchi can help maintain a healthy gut flora, which aids digestion and nutrient absorption. If you suspect you have a problem with nutrient absorption due to a health condition, consult a healthcare provider. They may recommend specific dietary changes or supplements to assist with this.
- **Enhance Bioavailability:** Certain food combinations can improve nutrient bioavailability. For example, consuming vitamin C-rich foods like oranges or bell peppers with iron-rich foods can enhance iron absorption. Similarly, fat-soluble vitamins A, D, E, and K are better absorbed when consumed with some dietary fat.
- **Monitoring Health Effects:** Regular health check-ups and blood tests can show how well your body utilizes nutrients and indicate potential deficiencies or excesses. For example, a comprehensive blood panel can show levels of vitamins, minerals, blood glucose, and cholesterol. Pay attention to how you feel, too. Changes in energy levels, mood, digestion, and physical appearance like skin, hair, and nails can all provide clues about your nutritional status.
- **Mindful Eating:** Pay attention to how your body responds to certain foods. Do you feel energized or sluggish after eating certain meals? Do some foods cause digestive discomfort? Listening to your body can provide valuable insights about what foods work best for you. Measuring nutrition is a comprehensive process involving careful observation, possibly some testing, and a mindful approach to eating. Remember, everyone is unique, so what works for one person may not work for another. It's all about finding what's best for your body and health. Begin with assessing your hydration.

Electrolytes and Hydration

Electrolytes, such as sodium, potassium, calcium, and others, play a critical role in maintaining homeostasis within the body. Electrolytes are essential minerals that play a vital role in many bodily functions, including:

- Regulating fluid balance
- Transmitting nerve impulses
- Contracting muscles
- Maintaining a healthy heart rhythm
- Building and maintaining bones and teeth
- Regulating blood pressure
- Converting food into energy
- Producing new cells
- Supporting the immune system

The main electrolytes in the body are sodium, potassium, calcium, magnesium, chloride, bicarbonate, and phosphate. Each electrolyte has a specific role in maintaining homeostasis, or balance, in the body. For example, sodium helps to regulate fluid balance, potassium helps to contract muscles, and calcium helps to build and maintain bones and teeth. Here is a breakdown:

- **Sodium:** The most abundant electrolyte in the body, sodium helps to regulate fluid balance and blood pressure. It is found primarily in the extracellular fluid, which is the fluid outside of cells.
- **Potassium:** The most abundant electrolyte inside cells, potassium helps regulate muscle contractions and nerve impulses. It is also involved in the metabolism of carbohydrates and proteins.
- **Calcium:** The most abundant mineral in the body, calcium is essential for building and maintaining bones and teeth. It is also involved in blood clotting, muscle contractions, and nerve impulses.
- **Magnesium:** A cofactor for over 300 enzymes, magnesium is involved in various bodily functions, including energy

production, protein synthesis, and nerve function. Many experts consider magnesium to be the number one most deficient mineral in most people.

- **Bicarbonate:** A buffer that helps maintain the pH balance of blood and other body fluids, bicarbonate is also involved in transporting carbon dioxide in the blood.
- **Phosphates:** Essential for energy storage and transfer, phosphates are also involved in the structure of DNA and RNA and bone formation.
- **Chloride:** The most abundant anion in the extracellular fluid, chloride helps to regulate fluid balance and blood pressure. It is also involved in the production of gastric acid.

Electrolytes play a vital role in many critical bodily functions. A disturbance in electrolyte balance can lead to various health issues, including dehydration, heart rhythm disturbances, muscle weakness, and more. Hence, maintaining a proper electrolyte balance is essential for the overall health and functioning of the human body.

Here's a basic table of the Recommended Dietary Allowances (RDAs) or Adequate Intake (AI) levels for some of the main electrolytes. The values for adults may vary depending on age, sex, physiological state (such as pregnancy), and individual health status.

Electrolyte	RDA/AI for Men	RDA/AI for Women
Sodium	1.5 g (AI)	1.5 g (AI)
Potassium	3.4 g (AI)	2.6 g (AI)
Chloride	2.3 g (AI)	2.3 g (AI)
Calcium	1.0 g	1.0 g

Magnesium	400-420 mg	310-320 mg
Phosphorus	700 mg	700 mg

Table 1 - Electrolyte Recommendations

Electrolytes and Keto

For someone following a Ketogenic or low-carb diet, it is often recommended to have between three and five grams of sodium per day as the lower intake of carbohydrates reduces the amount of sodium the body retains.

Electrolytes improve the transition to a ketogenic diet by helping to:

- **Reduce the risk of dehydration.** When you start a ketogenic diet, you may lose more fluids than usual through urination. This is because your body eliminates excess ketones by burning fat for energy. Electrolytes help to retain fluids in the body, which can help to prevent dehydration.
- **Prevent muscle cramps.** Muscle cramps are a common complaint among people transitioning to a ketogenic diet. This is because low electrolytes, such as potassium and magnesium, can contribute to muscle cramps. Getting enough electrolytes can help to prevent or relieve muscle cramps.
- **Improve energy levels.** When you start a ketogenic diet, you may experience fatigue or low energy levels. This is because your body is adjusting to using fat for energy instead of carbohydrates. Electrolytes help to improve energy levels by supporting the function of your nerves and muscles.
- **Reduce the risk of keto flu.** The keto flu is a group of symptoms that can occur when you start a ketogenic diet. These symptoms can include fatigue, headache, nausea, and muscle

cramps. Electrolyte deficiency is one of the leading causes of keto flu. Getting enough electrolytes can help to reduce the risk or severity.

Here are some tips for getting enough electrolytes on a ketogenic diet:

- Salt your food to taste. Many people have developed a habit of avoiding salt. On a Ketogenic diet, you should increase your daily salt intake by adding more to your food.
- Drink plenty of water with salt or electrolytes added. I recommend most people on a Keto diet avoid drinking plain water.
- Take electrolyte supplements, if necessary. Electrolyte supplements are available in powder, tablet, and liquid form.

If you are experiencing symptoms of dehydration, muscle cramps, or fatigue, it is crucial to increase your intake of electrolytes. You can do this by eating more electrolyte-rich foods, drinking more fluids, or taking electrolyte supplements. It is also important to note that everyone's electrolyte needs are different. Some people may need more electrolytes than others, depending on their activity level, diet, and overall health.

Electrolytes and Exercise

The role of sodium in enhancing athletic performance is closely tied to its ability to regulate hydration in the body. Hydration is a key performance factor, with even a modest loss of body water (as little as 2.5 percent weight loss) impairing the capacity to perform high-intensity exercise significantly. Therefore, focusing on hydration before exercise, known as preloading, can substantially improve performance.

The process of preloading involves consuming additional sodium with fluids before exercising. Sodium helps maintain blood volume, enabling optimal cardiovascular function and efficient dispersion of body heat. This, in turn, reduces fatigue and enables longer, sustained performance.

Preloading is particularly important because, during vigorous exercise, there is a substantial drop in blood plasma volume as the blood flows into your working muscles and skin, leaving less available for your cardiovascular system. By being fully hydrated beforehand, you have a larger reservoir of fluid to draw from, helping maintain blood volume and performance. Taking a sodium solution ninety minutes before exercise can boost performance, particularly in high-intensity, long-duration, or hot conditions. The recommended sodium concentration for this preload is 3,300 mg per liter of water, with a total fluid intake of twelve millileters per kilogram of body weight.

However, many athletes tend to under-hydrate, often starting their exercise sessions in a state of under-hydration. This decreases blood flow, sweat rates, and heat dissipation while increasing core temperature, resulting in inefficient energy use. Sodium is also critical in nutrient absorption, cognitive function, nerve impulse transmission, and muscle contraction.

While high sodium preloading can enhance performance, it is recommended for competitions or particularly strenuous exercise sessions rather than all intense training. Focusing on pre-hydration or preloading, especially with a high-sodium drink, can significantly enhance athletic performance. Post-workout hydration is also crucial for replenishing lost fluids and electrolytes, aiding recovery, and ensuring optimal performance in future workouts. However, testing your tolerance to high sodium preloading before a competitive event is essential to ensure it works for you.

Another topic of discussion when measuring nutrition is fasting. Common questions I hear often revolve around the benefits or detractors of eating at a particular time, how long an eating window should be, or the best way to break a fast. So, let's address it.

Fasting

It's important to consider ease of adherence, chance of adequate nutrition, and sustainability when deciding on a fasting protocol because they directly influence the success and health benefits you can receive from following any fasting plan.

No matter how beneficial a particular fasting protocol might be in theory, it won't be effective if it's too difficult for you to stick with it consistently. A regimen that aligns well with your daily routines, preferences, and lifestyle will be much easier to adhere to and is more likely to deliver the desired results.

Your body requires a wide range of nutrients to function optimally, including vitamins, minerals, protein, carbs, and fats. Getting the right balance of nutrients can be challenging when your eating window is limited. Inadequate nutrition can lead to deficiencies, which can have detrimental effects on your health, including impairing your immune system, slowing down your metabolism, and causing fatigue, among other issues.

Fasting protocols that are too extreme or challenging to maintain over the long term can lead to negative impacts, such as binge eating or developing unhealthy relationships with food. On the other hand, a sustainable protocol can be incorporated into your lifestyle for the long term, allowing you to reap the benefits continuously. Moreover, quick fixes often lead to quick rebounds in weight once the diet is stopped, whereas changes you can maintain over the long term can help sustain weight loss and health benefits.

For these reasons, it's crucial to consider these factors when choosing a fasting protocol. I will say it again: Everyone is different, and what works well for one person might not work well for another. It's also essential to consult with a healthcare professional before beginning any new diet or fasting regimen.

Fasting Method	Ease of Adherence	Chance of Adequate Nutrition	Sustainability
16/8 IF	7	8	8
OMAD	4	6	5
Extended Fasting	3	4	3

Tale 2 - Fasting Comparison

- **Ease of Adherence:** This measures how easy it is for the average person to stick with the diet. The 16/8 intermittent fasting (IF) method is generally considered the easiest to stick to because it mainly involves skipping breakfast, and eating in the afternoon and evening is more sociable and practical. OMAD and extended fasting are more challenging due to the longer fasting periods.

- **Chance of Adequate Nutrition:** The more frequently you eat, the easier it is to ensure you get all the nutrients your body needs. With 16/8 IF, there's still a decently-sized eating window to consume various foods. OMAD can make it more challenging to get adequate nutrition because you're trying to fit all your nutrients into one meal. Extended fasting is even more difficult because you're not consuming any food for an extended period.

- **Sustainability:** This measures how likely you are to maintain this method over a long period. Again, the 16/8 IF approach tends to be the most sustainable because it allows for a daily eating window. OMAD and extended fasting are less sustainable due to the restrictive nature of these methods.

It's crucial to understand that these are just rough estimates. To contextualize these topics, you must ask, "What's the goal?" Why go through the extra effort to force an eating pattern based on the clock? So, let's talk about that.

Benefits of Fasting

Fasting can have tremendous benefits and has a place in the toolbox. Several advantages to fasting include:

- **Autophagy:** Autophagy is a cellular process where cells recycle and renew their components. It helps to remove damaged proteins and organelles, fight infections, and adapt to stress. Fasting is a potent autophagy inducer and helps maintain cell function, homeostasis, and survival during starvation. It's associated with disease prevention and longevity.

- **Insulin Resistance:** Fasting can improve insulin sensitivity, making the body's cells more responsive to insulin. This can help with blood sugar control, which is especially beneficial for preventing and managing conditions like Type II diabetes.
- **Body Fat:** Fasting can lead to weight loss by helping you consume fewer fuel macros and enhancing hormone function to facilitate weight loss. It can increase levels of norepinephrine, which can enhance fat breakdown.
- **Mitochondrial Health:** Fasting can improve the health and function of the mitochondria, the energy-producing factories of our cells. This can lead to enhanced metabolic efficiency and overall better health and longevity.
- **Hormones:** Fasting influences numerous hormones. For example, it can increase human growth hormone levels, which helps with fat loss and muscle gain. It also affects insulin, ghrelin (the hunger hormone), and leptin (the satiety hormone), impacting appetite and energy use.
- **Appetite:** Fasting can help regulate the hormones involved with hunger and fullness, which can help with weight control. After an initial period, many people report decreased hunger and increased satisfaction with less food.
- **Immune System:** Fasting can help reduce inflammation and promote the regeneration of immune cells, which can lead to a more robust immune response. It can also trigger autophagy, which aids in maintaining immune system balance.
- **Improves BDNF (Brain-Derived Neurotrophic Factor):** BDNF is a protein that helps nerve cells grow, function, and survive. Fasting can boost levels of BDNF, which can have a protective effect on the brain and improve cognitive function.
- **Improves Cell Hormesis:** Hormesis refers to the beneficial effect of mild, transient stress—like that caused by fasting—on the body. It can enhance cellular defense, repair, and resistance, and can also increase the lifespan of cells.
- **Improves Metabolic Performance:** Fasting can improve various metabolic markers, such as cholesterol levels, blood glucose

levels, and insulin resistance. These benefits contribute to overall improved health and lower risk of chronic diseases like diabetes, heart disease, and certain cancers.

It's apparent why fasting is so popular. It has a lot of applications that can be used to improve many aspects of health. However, be wary of falling into the fasting trap. It is not a cure-all or a panacea for fixing all problems. Fasting has a place where it can be very effective, but it also needs to be stopped in favor of other methods when it's no longer working.

Fasting can be a great option to help you get your eating under control, retrain satiety signaling, lose body fat, and improve many factors of metabolic health. The downsides of fasting are its complexity, additional effort in planning, impact on lifestyle, and tendency to under-consume. Fasting is a great short-term tool that is too frequently overused and over-relied upon. Here's why.

Health First

Go back to the definition of health, and you see that fasting can help with pieces but not the whole picture. Fasting is focused on leveraging specific biological mechanisms to improve performance instead of providing a baseline of support to maintain performance. Fasting is a great way to get your body going in the right direction, but it doesn't make for a sound long-term solution.

Remember, the food you consume is like the gasoline that fuels a car, and exercise is like regularly taking your car out for a drive to ensure it continues to run smoothly. The car needs both a continuous supply of fuel and regular usage to maintain optimal performance.

Consider fasting as an engine cleaner or a booster additive you might put into your car. This additive helps clean the engine, improves fuel efficiency, and may enhance the vehicle's overall performance for a while. Similarly, fasting can 'clean up' our bodies through processes like autophagy, improve metabolic efficiency (like how a car might run better after an engine clean), and induce several beneficial physiological changes.

However, you can't continuously run your car on this additive alone. It's not meant to replace the fuel, nor is it a long-term substitute for regular usage and maintenance (exercise and a healthy lifestyle). If you kept trying to run the car only on the additive, you would eventually face problems because the car needs gasoline for its regular function.

So, in this analogy, fasting is a helpful tool for kickstarting certain biological processes and enhancing our body's efficiency and performance. Still, it's not a standalone solution for long-term health and well-being. Just like the car needs regular fuel and maintenance, our bodies need balanced nutrition and regular exercise to run smoothly over time.

The Whole Picture

The way to balance the impact of fasting is to include an exercise plan. A regular fitness routine will provide all the same benefits as fasting, with a boatload of additional ones fasting can never offer.

	Fasting	Exercise
Autophagy	Induces autophagy through nutrient deprivation	Stimulates autophagy due to the stress of physical activity
Insulin Resistance	Can improve insulin sensitivity by reducing fuel macro and carbohydrate intake	Increases insulin sensitivity by promoting glucose uptake into muscles
Body Fat	Can help reduce body fat through reduced fuel macro intake	Helps burn body fat by increasing energy expenditure
Mitochondrial Health	Induces autophagy, which aids in mitochondrial health and function	Improves mitochondrial function by creating more mitochondria in cells and activating mitophagy

Hormones	Can impact various hormones, e.g., increase human growth hormone levels	Stimulates the release of various hormones involved in metabolism, muscle growth, and mood regulation
Appetite	Can help to reset appetite regulation over a more extended period	Can suppress appetite in the short term
Immune System	Can reduce inflammation and promote the regeneration of immune cells	Moderate exercise can enhance immune function and stimulate the lymphatic system
Improves BDNF	Can increase levels of BDNF	Can also increase levels of BDNF
Improves Cell Hormesis	Causes mild stress, leading to cellular adaptations that will enhance health	Similar effects through the physical stress of exercise
Improves Metabolic Performance	Can improve metabolic health by influencing various markers such as cholesterol and blood glucose levels	Regular exercise helps maintain a lean mass, improve cardiovascular health, and reduce the risk of many chronic diseases
Improves Components of Fitness	N/A	Has a direct effect on all ten components of fitness
Improves Metabolic Flexibility	N/A	Enhances the ability to produce fuel and utilize the three pathways for energy
Improve Mobility and Functional Movement	N/A	Allows for developing and maintaining physical ability and freedom of movement

Table 3 - Fasting vs. Exercise

Fasting and fitness can be seen as two tools that, when used together strategically, can help optimize health and well-being.

In the early stages of someone's health program, fasting can serve as a powerful tool to kickstart weight loss, improve metabolic health, and create an initial spark of motivation. Fasting can induce rapid yet safe weight loss, help control blood sugar, reduce inflammation, and initiate processes such as autophagy, which help cleanse the body at a cellular level. This initial phase can be highly motivating for individuals, as they can often see and feel the benefits quite quickly.

However, fasting isn't a long-term solution. It's like a sprint at the beginning of a marathon – it gives a powerful start but cannot and should not be sustained for the entire race. Therefore, while fasting can be a helpful tool at the beginning and occasionally throughout someone's health program, it should be used selectively, with specific goals in mind, such as to break a weight-loss plateau or to induce autophagy.

On the other hand, fitness or regular physical exercise should form the backbone of any health program. Regular exercise improves cardiovascular health, strengthens muscles, enhances mobility, boosts mood, and promotes overall longevity. It's the tortoise in the race – consistent, dependable, and always moving forward.

As the individual progresses through their program and fasting phases become less frequent or stop, the base of physical fitness they've been building will ensure they continue to maintain and improve their health. Fitness helps build physical strength and endurance, improves flexibility and range of motion, and enhances balance and coordination. These improvements will translate into better daily function, increased energy levels, and a greater ability to engage in various physical activities.

While fasting can be an effective tool in certain stages or situations, fitness should always form the foundation of a health program. The benefits of regular physical exercise are vast and enduring, contributing to sustained health and well-being long after specific fasting interventions have ended.

Remember, it's a journey and not a destination. So, if you find yourself plateauing, you may need to consider upping your game to more advanced fitness concepts. Fitness is about conditioning the body and then challenging it in healthy ways.

Takeaways

- Inflammation is good until it's not
- Metabolic rate is a poor measure of overall health
- Macros are not relational. Adjust them individually based on results.
- Hydration requires more than water.
- Fast if you want. There migh be less complicated ways to reach your goals.

Resources

- Get **FREE** Bonus material that includes a complete breakdown and analysis of the most common fitness and nutrition programs to help you evaluate which ones will work best for you by following the F2 Method.
- Join **Coach Bronson's Body Confident Support Group** on Discord and meet more people who are improving themselves every day. https://discord.coachbronson.com
- Download the **FREE Body Confident Book Bonus Material** and Community information at https://bodyconfidentbook.com.

CHAPTER 10

- -

APPLYING THE F2 METHOD TO YOUR LIFE

"Knowledge without action is like having no knowledge at all!" - Ted Nichols

You are on a life-long journey. It ends when you die, not a moment sooner. The more you fight against this fact, the harder it will be for you to stay on track. You cannot look at the health improvement process with a short-term mindset. You need to view it through the lens of *"till death do us part."*

You need to realize and acknowledge that you've been on a health journey since birth. Your level of participation, intention, and control over where you're headed has been varied and inconsistent. Either you have done nothing or have been trying and haven't reached the lifestyle you're shooting for yet. Further, you may have ebbed and flowed from illness or injury and motivation or lack of motivation.

This is your reminder that any goals you set are just stepping stones along the path. There is no shortage of things you can do to improve your quality of life for years to come. Reaching a goal is not the end of your journey but the beginning of a new chapter in your story. There is no finish line where you can say you are done.

When you embrace a lifestyle of health, your perspective changes, and you begin to approach the process differently. You start to understand that health and well-being are not a destination but a life-long journey. It's about creating a lifestyle supporting your physical, mental, and emotional health, not achieving a temporary goal.

Instead of seeing the pursuit of health as a chore or obligation, you will find joy and satisfaction in it. This new perspective might mean finding physical activities you love, experimenting with healthy recipes, or learning to meditate. As you develop more enjoyment of the process, it becomes more sustainable. Decisions become easier because you are more connected to the long-term impacts of what health means to you.

When you acknowledge that there is no end date, you start thinking of possibilities for the future instead of expectations for the present. You understand there is no rush, and you have the rest of your life to work on yourself; there is much less stress. It's easier to get back on track, stay consistent, and move on after a setback.

Your health is your lifelong partner. Honor it with consistent care, attention, and commitment. It's not about being perfect; it's about making progress, one day at a time. You're not just improving your health; you're enhancing your quality of life. You're writing a story of resilience, self-care, and personal growth; every goal you achieve is a new, exciting chapter.

Apply Context and Perspective

Navigating your health journey can be like trying to find your way through a dense forest of information. Countless resources are available - books, social media posts, Google searches, podcasts, and more. All of these sources can provide valuable insights, but it's important to remember that not all information will be relevant or beneficial to your unique situation.

Understanding this begins with appreciating the power of perspective and context. Let's take the perspectives of a doctor and a coach, for example. A doctor may focus on immediate solutions to mitigate health risks - this is their perspective shaped by their medical training and goals of urgent patient care. The primary concern is to get you from a state of ill health to a state of stability as quickly as possible. In contrast, a coach may concentrate more on long-term strategies for physical improvement. They see your health journey as a marathon rather than a sprint, aiming to help you gradually increase your stamina, strength, or agility over time. This perspective is influenced by training in personal development and fitness, as well as a focus on gradual progress and lasting change. So, when you receive advice, it's crucial to consider the perspective of the person giving the guidance and the context in which they operate. What works in a medical context may not work in a fitness context, and vice versa.

Moreover, it's essential to recognize that there's no one-size-fits-all approach to health. What worked for someone else might not work for you because your body, lifestyle, goals, and health history are unique. It's not about finding a magic bullet but discovering what effectively supports your health and well-being.

Just as important is understanding that no single approach will always work. Your body changes as you age, and so do your health and fitness needs. What works for you now might not work five years down the line. Flexibility and adaptability are essential, as is a willingness to re-evaluate and adjust your approach.

While it's useful to absorb information from various sources, it's equally important to filter this information through the lens of your unique needs, context, and long-term goals. Being selective and patient with the process while maintaining an open mind can guide you to the strategies and habits that will best serve your health journey. Remember, it's not about what works for everyone else but what works for you.

Following the F2 Method

The F2 Method's core principles can help you interpret and apply the wealth of health information you encounter in your journey, ensuring it aligns with your needs. Here's how:

- **Prioritize Individual Goals:** When you come across new information or advice, consider how it aligns with your unique goals. Ask yourself if adopting this advice would move you closer to these goals or if it might distract or divert you from your path. Everyone's health journey is unique, so it's essential to tailor advice to your needs rather than mindlessly following general recommendations.

- **Get the Whole Picture:** Health and wellness are multifaceted, encompassing physical, mental, emotional, and environmental aspects. When you receive new information, consider how it fits into this broader perspective. For example, if a trendy diet ignores mental and emotional well-being, it may not be the right approach for you. Always remember to view health information in the context of your whole well-being.

- **Follow Concepts, Not Rules:** Health advice can often come across as rigid rules. But remember, what works for one person may not work for another. Use the underlying concepts as guidelines and adapt them to your unique situation. This approach fosters flexibility and personalization, allowing you to stay open to various methods and strategies to adapt to your individual health journey.

- **Make Solutions Sustainable:** You should consider any new health information or practices in the light of sustainability. Ask yourself if the suggested changes are feasible in the long term. If they seem too drastic or difficult to maintain, they might not be the best fit for your lifestyle.

- **Measure and Evaluate:** Keeping track of your progress is essential in determining what works for you. Whenever you try a new strategy, monitor its impact on your health. This evaluation will help you understand whether the new approach aligns with your health journey.

These five core concepts of the F2 Method can help you effectively evaluate health information from different perspectives, ensuring that it fits your individual context and goals.

Personalization, sustainability, and continuous measurement and evaluation are key in your health journey. The bottom line is that you are in this for the long haul. It is about the longevity of metabolic and physical freedom and not only improving your health but protecting it.

Become Body Confident

Improving your metabolic and physical freedom is the foundation for developing body confidence. When your body and mind are able to manage stress and your nutrition habits support optimal function, you gain a level of power and ability that changes the way you see and interact with the world.

- **Jenny C. 51 years old:** "My hunger is manageable again. I saw big gains in strength. I've added muscle, and I feel stronger. I've also learned that I am stronger and more capable than I thought. It's ok to be anxious about performing a movement, but my body has "got this!" The strength and confidence I've gained is unbelievable. My depression has lifted, I'm less stressed, sleep better, and I'm more hydrated and overall happier."

- **Theresa S. 52 years old:** "Recently I chaperoned the youth group from my church on a five mile hike on the Pacific Crest Trail. Not only did I do it, but I out-hiked some of the teenagers. In addition, the next day, I was in charge of the nursery at church and had to get up and down off the floor and play with the toddlers. And I was able to, with no problems."

- **Michelle H. 47 years old:** "I have a whole new understanding of what true health and fitness means. Not only am I stronger than I have ever been, but I am doing my best to reverse aging, so I am able to be an active and healthy woman approaching my fifties. I want to be a fit and fun grandma who does all the exciting stuff with the kids, one who wears them out rather than them wearing me out."

This is a very small sample of how your life can change when you follow the F2 Method. Being body confident looks different on everyone. How will it look on you?

CHAPTER 11

‒‒‒ ‒‒‒ ‒‒‒ ‒‒‒ ‒‒‒ ‒‒‒ ‒‒‒ ‒‒‒ ‒‒‒ ‒‒‒ ‒‒‒ ‒‒‒ ‒‒‒ ‒‒‒ ‒‒‒ ‒‒‒ ‒‒‒ ‒‒‒ ‒‒‒ ‒‒‒

60 DAYS TO BODY CONFIDENT

"Anyone who has never made a mistake has never tried anything new." ~ Albert Einstein

Now you've read all this information, what do you do with it? You've learned about the core concepts and principles that build the foundation you need to improve your quality of life. How do you take those ideas and put them into practice?

You need a blueprint, something to help you step by step, day by day, practice and learn how to apply the F2 Method in your everyday life. That is what this chapter is all about.

The goal of this sixty day program is to walk you through the process of finding your why, setting some goals, and identifying what the most attainable and sustainable steps you need to take are to move you in the right direction.

If you do this correctly, it will be uniquely yours. No one will have the same experience, because no one will do it the same way as anyone else.

How it works

The 60 Days to Body Confident program is eight weeks long. There are three phases that match directly to the Quality of Life Domains (Mindset, Fitness, and Nutrition)

The first two weeks are your opportunity to find your Why, understand your Context, and define a Vision for your life.

The next three weeks are where you start making small changes in your nutrition to support long-term success and metabolic freedom.

The final three weeks will focus on developing habits to support the principles of fitness that will create true physical freedom in your life.

Each phase builds on the next. If you pay attention and really focus, you can follow this process indefinitely and continue your journey well past sixty days.

Before you get started

There are a four actions you need to take to get the most out of the next sixty days. If you're serious about finding the best path forward, do these things first. If you don't, the next sixty days will be a waste of your time.

1. **Find at least one person to do this with or get support from.** A handful of close friends is even better. No one is perfect. Everyone needs support in their journey. Accountability and sharing this challenge with someone adds a significant chance that you will be more successful over the next sixty days.

   Whether it's a 60 Days to Body Confident partner or just a friend that will help you stay on track and maintain an environment for you to make good choices, every bit of support is a bonus to your progress. Stay in regular contact, talk, share, and vent with each other. Most importantly, remind yourself and your partner of WHY you dicided to do this and keep the emotion of that feeling at the front of your mind at all times.

   Meet other members participating in the 60 Day program on our dedicated Discord server at http://bodyconfidentbook.com.

2. **Define your obstacles ahead of time.** Do not start the program until you have written down a list of things that you think will make it challenging. The next sixty days are not going to be easy. The things you're going to do, are new and outside your comfort zone.

Whether it's work, your family schedule, or upcoming events, you must prepare yourself for the times when your mind will try and trick you into quitting. Make a plan and decided how you are going to change your environment or succeed within it. You already the know the things that you let yourself make excuses for. Stop it before it even happens.

3. **Stop looking for the "Right" answer.** The whole reason for this book and this program is to help you set expectations and experiment to find the best solution for you. I can't tell you what's best for you. I can help you find a starting point and give you directions on how to move forward from there. The F2 Method is a map, not a rule book.

   If someone is telling you what to do, then it won't be your individual solution.

What You Need to Do

The challenge is broken up into three phases to walk you through the F2 Method and help you make decisions and set goals that are attainable over the next eight weeks. First, let's review the F2 Method then get into how the challenge works and what you ended to do next.

F2 Method Review

Before you get deep into the challenge, review what the F2 Method is and how you will use it to build your personalized quality of life plan.

The F2 Method is a holistic evaluation of an individual's lifestyle, environment, and goals, using an understanding of evidence-based health concepts and principles to build a sustainable plan that measurably improves your quality of life.

The F2 Method presents a unique framework for lifestyle planning, emphasizing personalization and sustainability. It is designed to facilitate successful lifestyle changes by focusing on individual needs and goals.

Central to the F2 Method are five core concepts that serve as the foundation for navigating the vast landscape of health information and translating it into sustainable actions. These concepts are:

1. **Prioritize Individual Goals:** Tailoring plans to personal aspirations.
2. **Get the Whole Picture:** Considering all aspects of a situation.
3. **Follow Concepts, Not Rules:** Embracing flexibility over rigidity.
4. **Make Solutions Sustainable:** Focusing on long-term applicability.
5. **Measure and Evaluate:** Continuously assessing progress.

The F2 Method extends its influence through three primary domains of Quality of Life: Mindset, Fitness, and Nutrition. Each domain is crucial in building a holistic approach to health and well-being.

8 WEEK SCHEDULE

NOTES
Each week builds on the next. Whatever you do in one week, keep doing it as you add the next week's goal.

GET READY
1. Get support
2. Define your obstacles
3. Reset your expectations

PHASE 1
WEEKS 1 AND 2 - MINDSET
1. Find your WHY
2. Clarify what you don't want
3. Decide who you want to be
4. Set your goals

PHASE 2
WEEKS 3 TO 5 - NUTRITION
1. Improve your Nutrient Density
2. Focus on Bioavailability
3. Eat more satiating options

PHASE 3
WEEKS 6 TO 8 - FITNESS
1. Focus on Proper Movement
2. Increase training resistance
3. Be more consistent

MEASURE AND ADJUST
DON'T STOP
This process repeats over and over. At regular intervals, you need to evaluate your progress and make adjustments that move you closer to your long-term goals.

1. **Mindset Domain:** Encompasses self-awareness, future vision, identity, beliefs, and habits.
2. **Fitness Domain:** Focuses on the body's performance, recovery, and stress management.

3. **Nutrition Domain:** Involves body functionality, efficiency, and internal stress management.

Each Quality of Life Domain is guided by three specific tenets, making up a total of nine tenets. These tenets are essential for ensuring balanced and comprehensive progress.

- **Tenets One Through Three (Mindset)**
    - Know Why
    - Know You
    - Know How
- **Tenets Four Through Six (Fitness)**
    - Move Well
    - Move Weight
    - Move Often
- **Tenets Seven Through Nine (Nutrition)**
    - Nutrient Density
    - Bioavailability
    - Satiety

60 Day to Body Confident Schedule

I'm not going to tell you how to do everything over the next sixty days. The reason for this challenge is for you to accept responsibility for your results. That means you have to ask your own questions, evaluate your own responses, and make your own choices.

This sixty day program is your guide. It doesn't have all the answers. Those are yours to figure out.

Phase 1 (Weeks 1 and 2) - Mindset

The first two weeks are not for you to make any changes in your nutrition or fitness activities. Use this time to get your mind ready for success. If you skip this phase or don't really put the effort in, the rest of this process is going to be a struggle.

If you really put yourself into this phase, the next two phases will be a walk in the park and you will see more success over these eight weeks than you ever thought possible.

Over the next two weeks, I want you to spend time, every day working through these four questions and activities.

- Why are you doing this? This is your "Why"
- What are you trying to avoid? This is your "Why Not"
- Who do you want to be? This is your vision
- How are you going to get there? This is your goal.

Why are you doing it? - Know Your Why

The most important question you can ask yourself is, "Why am I doing this?" I'm not talking about losing ten pounds, getting back to your pre-baby weight, or even because your doctor said you need to. I'm talking about knowing what the changes you want to make will do for your everyday life and their impact on you and everyone in your life.

Your decision to get healthy has a much bigger impact than just losing some weight. What does it mean to you? How will your life change? What will you be able to do? Who will you inspire, and what kind of example will your effort provide for others?

Getting out of shape doesn't come by accident. It is a deliberate action, repeatedly producing a result. The law of inertia means that it will take MORE deliberate action with MORE consistency to reverse the momentum of your fitness and health and start moving in a positive direction.

When you're at the movies and the smell of popcorn and sight of people eating French fries and candy is all around you, your reason for staying true to your goals must be larger than the temptations around you.

The only thing that will keep you going is knowing why you're doing it. Your "why" has to be bigger than your "but."

Finding your "Why"

No one wakes up in the morning and randomly decides to lose weight. Losing weight is a goal many people use after years of mental or physical trauma caused by poor health and physical ability. People want to lose weight due to feeling worthless, lack of independence, chronic pain, and illness. There is always a bigger reason than the weight itself.

You don't want to lose weight. You want what you think losing weight will do for your quality of life and mental health. It's the effect on how you live every day that matters, not how much you weigh.

Here are some signs that you've dug deep enough and found the real reason you want to change your life.

- You can't think about it without getting emotional. When you find your "Why" it will make you angry, sad, give you hope, or fire you up! You shouldn't be able to have an unemotional conversation about your "Why."
- Nothing is too inconvenient. The things you thought would be a challenge won't be nearly as tough. When you are in touch with your "Why," you don't let anything stand in your way.
- You won't hear the noise. People don't like change. Many people in your life will try and keep you where you are. Not everyone is ready to do what you're doing. When you have a solid reason that drives you forward, no one will be able to stop you.

Activity - The 7 Levels of Why

Here is an exercise you can do to help get to the real reason you've started this journey. Be honest with yourself. No one is watching but you. You are going to have resistance, that's normal. Pushing through that self-limitation is the only way you're going to be successful long-term

NOTE: This is NOT a five-minute exercise. It may take you a week to get through this. Dig deep, and don't let fear or embarrass- ment hold you back.

Ask yourself "Why" at least seven times, using the answer each time as the subject of the next question. Example:

- **Q.** "Why am I doing this challenge?"
- **A.** "I'm doing this challenge because I want to lose weight."
- **Q.** "Why do I want to lose weight?"
- **A.** "I want to lose weight because I will feel more confident in myself if I was twenty-five pounds lighter."
- **Q.** "Why does my confidence rely on me weighing a certain amount?"

......Keep going until you get all in your feels.

If you're struggling with identifying your "Why," start looking at the things you've been using as excuses for not doing what you know you should.

Your excuses are just your reasons in disguise.

- "I don't have time," is really, "I want to get better at organizing my life."
- "I'm too old." is really, "I want to get healthy to be more independent as I get older."
- "I'm not a gym person." is really, "I want to be an active person and improve my physical ability."

Every single excuse you can make is a reason you need to take action to improve your life!

The Cost of Comfort

What happens if you do NOT change course, not just in one year, but in five years?

The goal here, even though it may feel unpleasant, is to construct a very detailed and specific picture of what the future may hold. A foreshadowing of things to come if you don't change. Imagine where you might find yourself not just next year, but in five years, if you do not change your current lifestyle. This exercise, though challenging, is essential for envisioning what could be, if you choose to embrace change.

Our instincts often resist change, interpreting it as a threat to our safety and comfort. This is like a person staying in a dimly lit, familiar room, avoiding the sunlight outside because it's unfamiliar and seemingly intense. In your health journey, this room represents your current habits—perhaps sedentary behavior or unhealthy eating—which, while familiar, might not be beneficial to your long-term well-being.

Stepping out of this room, though initially uncomfortable due to the blinding light, is akin to adopting new, healthier habits. It's a venture into the unknown, which naturally feels risky.

However, just as our eyes adjust to sunlight, revealing a vibrant world outside, your body and mind can adapt to healthier habits, unveiling a life of improved health and vitality.

The benefits of this change are substantial. Picture a future where you have embraced these new habits: increased energy, better health, a sense of achievement. This isn't just about avoiding negative outcomes; it's about moving towards a positive, vibrant future.

REMEMBER: Embracing change in your health habits can lead to a positive transformation over the next five years, while staying in your comfort zone is likely to result in a decline in health and well-being.

Feeling a bit of fear or discomfort during this exercise is normal and even beneficial. It's a sign that you are confronting the realities of what might happen if you don't change. The key is to focus on the brighter, healthier future that awaits you if you dare to step out of your comfort zone.

Activity - Define what do you want to avoid

This exercise is not just an intellectual activity; it's a powerful tool for change. If you're hesitant to engage in it for fear of feeling uneasy, consider how much more challenging it would be to face the real consequences of inaction in five years. It's far more advantageous to confront these feelings now, in a controlled and constructive way, than to experience them as your lived reality later on.

Answer the following questions in as much specific detail as you can. If you don't make any changes in your habits or lifestyle...

- What will happen to my confidence and how, specifically, will this negatively impact my life?
- What specific negative changes in my physical condition will I experience? Be detailed.
- What specific health concerns would be worse compared to today? How much worse? Would I have any NEW health concerns that I don't have today?
- How might my energy and/or fatigue level change for the worse? What specific negative impact will that have in my life as compared to today?
- How might my relationships suffer as compared today? *Include the specific negative impact on colleagues, friends, peers, children, spouse, and family.*
- How might I need to dress differently as compared today? *Include the specific clothing choices you'd have to make and/or could no longer make.*
- How might my career and/or finances have been negatively impacted? Look carefully and detail the difference below. *If you DO see a difference in your financial and/or career activities, try to QUANTIFY how much of a financial impact there might be in five years if you don't change.*
- What negative changes in my physical ability, sports participation, and/or activity level do I see five years from now if I don't change course?

Now, review your answers above and record the most motivating negative consequences. Again, we're trying to discern what is most motivating for you. Some people are hyper-focused on just a few motivators, while others may have a dozen or more. There is no good or bad. Your motivators are your motivators!

Identifying the things we want to avoid is a crucial aspect of motivation because it helps to create a clear contrast between our current path and the potential negative outcomes of inaction. By vividly understanding what we wish to steer clear of, whether it's poor health, unfulfilled potential, or any other undesirable situation, we gain a powerful impetus to change. This awareness acts as a catalyst, pushing us beyond complacency and towards positive action. It's not just about fear of the negative; it's about recognizing the full spectrum of possibilities and consciously choosing a path that leads us away from what we don't want and towards what we do. This approach helps to solidify our goals, provides a sense of urgency, and keeps us aligned with our desired future.

Build a vision of your future - Know You

Establishing your new identity is a deeply personal and transformative process. It's about discovering who you are at your core – your values, beliefs, passions, and the roles you play in your social circles. Think of it as developing your unique internal compass, one that guides you through life's complexities, offering direction and purpose. This process of self-discovery isn't just a moment of introspection; it's an ongoing dialogue with yourself, shaped by your experiences, relationships, and aspirations.

By actively engaging in this journey, you start to piece together a coherent picture of yourself. It involves looking inward to understand your strengths, acknowledging your weaknesses, and embracing the unique qualities that make you, you. This isn't a static process – your identity evolves as you grow and encounter new experiences. It's like crafting your life's narrative, a story that's uniquely yours. Having a strong sense of who you are brings a host of benefits: it boosts your confidence, builds resilience, and enriches your relationships. A well-defined identity allows you to connect with others more authentically, as you interact from a place of self-awareness and truth. So, as you navigate this path, remember that establishing your identity is not just about finding yourself – it's about creating who you wish to be, a beautiful and ever-evolving journey.

As you define a new identity and envision your future self, you're setting the stage for a transformative journey. This vision acts as a blueprint, outlining not just who you want to become, but also the actions and habits that characterize your future self. It's like painting a detailed portrait of the person you aspire to be – perhaps more confident, healthier, more successful, or more balanced. This portrait includes not just the traits you want to develop, but also the behaviors and routines that these traits embody.

Once you have this vision, you can start to emulate the actions and habits of your future self in your current life. For instance, if your future self is a successful entrepreneur, what habits does that person have? Are they disciplined, creative, a lifelong learner? If you see your future self as fit and healthy, what daily routines would they follow? This is where the power of your vision comes into play. By acting 'as if' you are already that person, you begin to instill the habits and behaviors that will eventually mold you into that identity.

This approach is like reverse engineering your life. **You're not waiting to become that person to start doing those things; you're doing those things to become that person.** It's a proactive and dynamic process. Each action you take is a step closer to that envisioned future. It might feel a bit unnatural or challenging at first, like trying on a new outfit that doesn't quite fit yet. But with time, these actions and habits will feel more natural, becoming an integral part of who you are.

This method is not just about dreaming of a future self; it's about living it in the present, making it a reality through consistent practice and commitment. Remember, every great journey starts with a single step, and each step you take in emulating your future self brings you closer to realizing that vision for your life.

Activity - Establish a vision and identity (3 steps)

The purpose of this exercise is to reprogram your subconscious mind and slowly make a shift towards becoming the best version of yourself. It's important that you revisit this exercise and vision often because repetition is the secret ingredient to make this exercise effective.

1. Character Traits

Write down five character traits you feel that you will need in order to be successful in your efforts to improve your health and have more freedom. Include what that character trait means to you.

Examples:

- Consistent - I am consistent in keeping my schedule for going to the gym.
- Self- Aware - I pay attention to my emotions and triggers.
- Frugal - I am smart with money.
- Organized - I focus on planning.
- Thick Skinned - I am not afraid of criticism.
- Empowering - I empower and enable others.
- Honest - I don't lie to myself or others.
- Beginner's Mindset - I ask for help when I need it.
- Humble - I lead without arrogance.
- Strategic - I plan ahead, don't act first.
- Visionary - I get people to buy into my vision.
- Attentive - I hear what people are saying between the lines.
- Courageous - I am not afraid to speak the truth.
- All In - I have a whatever it takes mentality.

2. Beliefs

Write down 5 beliefs that you will need to have in order to reprogram your mental filter and how you see the world. These beliefs will provide context for everything that happens to you and how you handle situations. Examples:

- I am a good mother and I set a great example for my kids.
- The results I get are directly related to the effort I put in.
- Speaking the truth builds trust in myself and others.
- Having a plan is the best way to succeed.
- Not everyone will agree with me and that's OK.
- I'm not trying to be like anyone else.
- I'm patient and willing to do things the right way.

3. Vision

Using the character traits and beliefs that you want to have, I want you to create a story. This story is about a future version of yourself. The person you aspire to be. You MUST set aside all reservations and THINK BIG!!!

Be as detailed as possible. Don't limit what this person's life could look like. Put your deepest dreams and desires into it. To get started, ask yourself:

- What does this person do everyday?
- What habits do they keep in their lives?
- What have they let go of to get where they are?
- What do they do to improve themselves regularly?
- What limitations have they overcome and how did they do it?
- How often do they spend time doing self-care and recovery?
- What is their relationship with their spouse?
- Who is this person, how do they live, interact with people, and spend their time?
- What have they accomplished and how does fitness and health affect their life?

Write this in the third person. You are creating a profile of someone you are trying to emulate. Imagine yourself on the outside looking in.

Example (please don't just copy this):

Bronson Dant is a successful entrepreneur, thought leader, and trend-setter. He is famous for reforming and leading a global health movement, making it possible for people all over the world to rediscover their self-confidence and personal freedom through improving their minds and bodies. His F2 Method has changed the health industry and become a movement - a paradigm that teaches people how to empower themselves and live life to its fullest.

Bronson is responsible for teaching people how to be balanced, integrated, and inspiring leaders who lead society to a new era of higher personal freedom. Anyone that learns from him becomes powerful beyond measure because they learn to master themselves. He has a vision to help people. His method has changed the way society fundamentally behaves and perceives reality.

Bronson lives on a beach, in a modern, technologically advanced home. It overlooks the ocean and mountains, and at night, you can see every star and constellation. In the evenings, he loves to sit in the open air and spend time with his partner around a cozy fire, in the hot tub, or on the beach. He spends the mornings preparing for the day to the sound of the ocean and works with a calm, grounded, relentless energy - no matter what's put in his way. Bronson lets stress roll off his back like it's nothing. He knows there is nothing to worry about because he knows what he's made of.

Bronson also knows how to have a good time! He brings the party wherever he goes, making each moment rich with playfulness and infectious optimism. Nobody can mess with his groove. He drives an Audi RS 5 but rolls low-key in a Jeep Grand Cherokee Trackhawk 4x4.

Bronson works out every day either with friends in his home gym or at a local gym. Bronson is a scratch bowler who enjoys several games in a league each week. In his beach home, he spends his evenings learning to play the drums, shooting on his private shooting range, and reading books, or writing his own.

If your vision isn't big, is it worth having?

As you develop this vision and answer these questions, you will create your path forward and the actions you need to take to bring this vision to life.

Setting Goals - Know How

In Chapter Seven I discussed a lot of topics in the Mindset domain. Goal setting is one of them. Here is a repeat of that information. This time, I want you to take some action and create your own goals following the framework I provide.

Recommendation for the next sixty days

I recommend you use this section to set your goals for the next sixty days. You can follow the process and get some practice setting goals. Use the steps to determine how you are going to meet the challenge for the nutrition and fitness aspects for the rest of the challenge. This is a great way to get experience setting goals that you can use even after the challenge is over.

Activity - Set your goals

Goals give you a direction to aim for and can help you maintain focus on your priorities. Without them, you might drift aimlessly without making meaningful progress in any specific area. Goals help you effectively channel your energy and resources toward achieving desired outcomes. They give you a way to track and gauge your progress.

Be S.M.A.R.T

To make sure your goals are clear and reachable, each one should be:

- Specific (simple, sensible, significant).
- Measurable (meaningful, motivating).
- Achievable (agreed, attainable).

- **R**elevant (reasonable, realistic and resourced, results-based).
- **T**ime-bound (time-based, time-limited, time/cost limited, timely, time-sensitive).

S.M.A.R.T. goals require you to define precisely what you want to achieve. This clarity removes ambiguity and provides a clear direction for your efforts. Instead of having a vague goal like "get fit," a specific goal would be "run a 5K in under thirty minutes."

SPECIFIC: Your goal should be clear and specific. Otherwise, you won't focus your efforts or feel truly motivated to achieve it. When drafting your goal, try to answer the five "W" questions:

- What do I want to accomplish?
- Why is this goal important?
- Who is involved?
- Which resources or limits are involved?

For example: I want to build muscle mass and improve my strength.

MEASURABLE: Having measurable goals to track your progress and stay motivated is essential. Assessing progress helps you stay focused, meet your deadlines, and feel the excitement of getting closer to achieving your goal. How will you know when you've reached the goal? A measurable goal should address questions such as:

- How much?
- How long?
- How fast?
- How heavy?

For example: I want to build five pounds of muscle mass and improve my strength to squat my body weight one time.

ACHIEVABLE: Your goal must also be realistic and attainable to succeed. In other words, it should stretch your abilities but remain possible. When you set an achievable goal, you may identify previously overlooked opportunities or resources that can bring you closer to it. An attainable goal will usually answer questions such as:

- How can I accomplish this goal?

- How realistic is the goal, based on other constraints, finances, or work schedule?

For example: I want to build five pounds of muscle mass and improve my strength to squat my body weight one time. I will do this by resistance training three times a week and eating one time my lean body mass in grams of protein daily.

Tip: Make sure you are setting goals for yourself. Don't be persuaded into saying you want to accomplish something just to make someone else happy or fulfill what you think someone else's desire for you is. Find out what excites you about your new life and go in that direction.

RELEVANT: This step ensures that your goal matters to you and aligns with other relevant goals. We all need support and assistance in achieving our goals, but it's crucial to retain control over them. So, ensure that your plans drive everyone forward but that you're still responsible for achieving your goal. A relevant goal can answer "yes" to these questions:

- Does this seem worthwhile?
- Will this goal have a positive impact on my life?
- Does this match other efforts/needs?

For example: I want to build five pounds of muscle mass and improve my strength to squat my body weight one time. I will do this by resistance training three times a week and eating one time my lean body mass in grams of protein per day. Doing this will improve my daily energy and reduce my back pain.

TIME-BOUND: Every goal needs a target date, a deadline to focus on, and something to work toward. This part of the SMART goals criteria prevents everyday tasks from taking priority over your longer-term goals. A time-bound goal will usually answer these questions:

- When?
- What can I do six months from now?
- What can I do six weeks from now?
- What can I do today?

For example: In the next six months, I want to build five pounds of muscle mass and improve my strength to squat my body weight one time.

I will do this by resistance training three times a week and eating one time my lean body mass in grams of protein daily. Doing this will improve my daily energy and reduce my back pain.

Now that's a goal you can build a solid plan from. What will your first goal be?

In case you weren't paying attention, the effort you have to put into your intention, expectations, belief systems, and building your identity is most of the work. The biggest mistake people make is thinking that their health journey is all about food and fitness. It's not. Your mind is where the power lies. Your success is 100% dependent on your willingness to change how you think about yourself and the world around you.

Using The F2 Method to Set Goals

Setting goals is not only a process of deciding what you're going to do, but figuring out what you CAN do, are WILLING to do, and are ABLE to do. This is where the F2 Method helps the most.

Every decision or goal should be weighed against the five core concepts of the F2 Method.

Is the goal you are setting for yourself:

- specific to your desires and context"
- considering as many lifestyle factors as possible?
- based on the minimum effective change that will help you see results?.
- something that you are willing and able to do long-term?
- something you can measure and quantify its achievement?

If you can't answer "yes" to each of these, it's likely that you will be less successful in accomplishing that goal.

Setting Your Sixty Day Goals

Before you finish Phase 1 - Mindset, and move into Phase 2 - Nutrition, you need to set your goals for the Nutrition and Fitness phases of the challenge. I'll walk you through the process. Once you have your goals, the rest of the challenge is all about execution. You are making all the decisions here, before you move on. **After this is done, you don't have to make the decisions again, you just have to follow-through.**

Your goals for Phases in the next six weeks need to meet the following requirements:

- only add one thing per week
- each week builds on the previous week
- each goal MUST meet all five Core Concepts of the F2 Method
- each goal can only be for the specific Tenet of that week

Each week, you focus on adding one thing to your routine or lifestyle. Whatever you add for your first nutrition goal, keep doing it for the whole challenge. the following week, your next goal will be added for the rest of the challenge as well. By the end of the program, you will have six new habits that you've started building into your life.

Weekly Goals

I'm going to use **Week 3 - Nutrient Density** to demonstrate the format that you will use each week as you build your new habits and lifestyle.

Week 3 - Nutrient Density (EXAMPLE)

This week I will increase the amount of nutrition in my food by, _increasing the amount of red meat I eat by eight ounces per day._

Is this goal:

- specific to your desires and context _(Yes, I want to get more nutrition and increase my protein intake)_
- considering as many lifestyle factors as possible? _(Yes, adding two to four more ounces of red meat per meal or even just one additional serving per day allows me to keep my current_

eating schedule and actually helps me feel fuller without snacking all day.)

- based on the minimum effective change that will help you see results? *(Yes, I think I am under-eating red meat and even as little amount as eight ounces per day will help build the habit and get my body used to larger amounts in the future.)*
- something that you are willing and able to do long-term? *(Yes, this is doable and doesn't seem like it will be to hard to do.)*
- something you can measure and quantify its achievement? *(Yes, if I measure and track it.)*

Follow this process for each of the areas you are going to set goals for the remainder of challenge. You can reference earlier sections of this book to refresh yourself on what the intention and impact of each tenet is and how you can approach small changes over the next few weeks.

Fill out your goals in the following sections so you know what you are doing over the next 6 weeks.

Phase 2 (Weeks 3 to 5) - Nutrition

What are your goals for the next three weeks? Remember, start with Nutrient Density, then add in Bioavailability next week, while continuing to meet your Nutrient Density goal. Keep the five core concepts of the F2 Method in mind and make sure the goals you set are achievable and sustainable.

Week 3 - Nutrient Density
This week I will increase the amount of nutrition in my food by,

_____

Is this goal:

- specific to your desires and context?
- considering as many lifestyle factors as possible?
- based on the minimum effective change that will help you see results?
- something that you are willing and able to do long-term?
- something you can measure and quantify its achievement?

Common goals reference:

- increase red meat intake by eight ounces.
- switch from sodas to water with electrolytes
- add an extra egg to one meal a day
- stop snacking and eat full meals three times a day

Week 4 - Bioavailability

This week I will increase the bioavailability of my food by,

Is this goal:

- specific to your desires and context?
- considering as many lifestyle factors as possible?
- based on the minimum effective change that will help you see results?
- something that you are willing and able to do long-term?
- something you can measure and quantify its achievement?

Common goals reference:

- stop using seed oils and start using animal fat
- replace processed/plant-based creamers with butter or real cream
- eat less raw and more fermented veggies
- choose fattier meat options

Week 5 - Satiety

This week I will increase the amount of satiety I get from my food by,

Is this goal:

- specific to your desires and context?
- considering as many lifestyle factors as possible?
- based on the minimum effective change that will help you see results?
- something that you are willing and able to do long-term?
- something you can measure and quantify its achievement?

Common goals reference:

- eat three meals a day
- eat protein on my plate first
- increase portions at each meal
- eat the whole food instead of a processed alternative

Phase 3 (Weeks 6 to 8) - Fitness

What are your goals for the last three weeks of the rest of your life? Remember, start with Moving Well, then add in Moving Weight next week, while continuing to meet your Moving Well goal. Keep the five core concepts of the F2 Method in mind and make sure the goals you set are achievable and sustainable.

Week 6 - Move Well

This week I will improve the quality of my movement by,

Is this goal:

- specific to your desires and context?
- considering as many lifestyle factors as possible?
- based on the minimum effective change that will help you see results?
- something that you are willing and able to do long-term?
- something you can measure and quantify its achievement?

Common goals reference:

- doing at least three full range of motion warm-up sets before I start my workout
- only increase weight or reps if I can do the current weight or reps multiple weeks in a row
- identify one range of motion limitation and work on it at least three times week
- record my movement and have a coach review it each week

Week 7 - Move Weight

This week I will increase the resistance or intensity of my workouts by,

---

Is this goal:

- specific to your desires and context?
- considering as many lifestyle factors as possible?
- based on the minimum effective change that will help you see results?
- something that you are willing and able to do long-term?
- something you can measure and quantify its achievement?

Common goals reference:

- adding more weight to the exercise (after consistent performance)
- making the exercise more complex (seated squat to a full squat)
- add an additional set or reps to the workout
- progress from an assisted to unassisted exercise

Week 8 - Move Often

This week I will increase consistency in moving my body by,

Is this goal:

- specific to your desires and context?
- considering as many lifestyle factors as possible?
- based on the minimum effective change that will help you see results?
- something that you are willing and able to do long-term?
- something you can measure and quantify its achievement?

Common goals reference:

- going to the gym three times per week
- not taking the elevator
- parking as far from the store as I can
- going for a fifteen minute walk after dinner

Measuring and Adjusting

As you go through the next few weeks, you need to be tracking how well you are accomplishing your goals. Are you goals performance based, meaning you either did the thing or you didn't? Are they results based, meaning you either hit the goal or you didn't? Either way, how are you tracking it?

Other things to measure

Besides tracking and measuring the specific actions and results of your goals, what about the other things that are impacted by improving your mindset, nutrition, and fitness? Have you gained muscle, lost fat, stopped feeling worn down, have a more positive attitude? What things are getting better?

Many people start this process looking at one or two things they want to improve. Luckily following the F2 Method had given you a lot more you can look at to see how you're doing.

Go back and look at the earlier chapters in the book. There are ten components to fitness, seven essential movements and three metabolic pathways. Just on the fitness side of your health, that makes twenty-one things where you can objectively measure improvement.

The impact of making changes to your nutrition can be seen in all sorts of biological and neurological aspects of your health. Body composition, mood, stress, energy, not to mention bloodwork, symptoms of illness and dysfunction are areas you can look at to find improvement in your quality of life.

Making Adjustments

The first thing to realize is that you can't make adjustments if you don't know what to adjust. Refer back to the Chapter 7 section titled, "If you're not tracking you're not trying." Remember that small adjustments work best. Just like when you set goals, be honest with yourself about what you are READY, WILLING, and ABLE to do. Most of all be patient.

What happens after Sixty Days?

Learning and building habits doesn't end after sixty days.

The whole idea is to help you learn how to use the F2 Method and continue the process by repeating it at your own pace throughout the rest of your life. The principles of the F2 Method are timeless and no matter where you are in your journey they are the path to get you where you want to go.

At the end of the sixty days, ask yourself;

- What went well?
- What did I struggle with?
- What did I achieve?
- What changes did I see in my life and health?
- What felt easy to me?
- What would I do differently next time?
- How could I make it more realistic?

Take all of those answers and use them to start 60 Days to Body Confident again!

Remember, you're on this journey for the rest of your life. Do you want to drive the car, or are you just along for the ride?

Download the FREE Body Confident Bonus Material at https://bodyconfidentbook.com

What's Next?

The principles of the F2 Method are timeless, and no matter where you are in your journey they are the path to get you where you want to go. This book took you far, but the learning doesn't end here. Download all the FREE Body Confident Bonus Material at https://bodyconfidentbook.com

REFERENCES

Jenkinson, C. (2023, February 28). quality of life. Encyclopedia Britannica. https://www.britannica.com/topic/quality-of-life

Dant B K, Changes in body composition and physical performance in peri and post-menopausal women following a ketogenic diet and functional fitness program. J Nutr Metab Health Sci 2022;5(3):124-128, https://www.jnmhs.com/article-details/17344

ABOUT THE AUTHOR

Bronson Dant is a health and fitness coach who has committed over a decade to guiding and training people in their pursuit of body confidence. With a fervor for physical activity and a desire to positively impact others, Bronson's journey toward a fulfilling career in fitness took an exciting turn when he discovered CrossFit around his fortieth birthday.

From the moment Bronson was introduced to CrossFit, he fell in love with its dynamic nature, vibrant community, effective coaching techniques, and transformative results. It became clear to him that delving deeper into the realm of fitness and becoming a coach was the natural progression for his life's path.

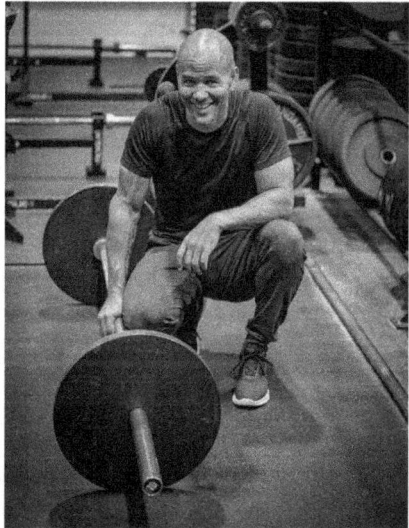

In 2014, Coach Bronson realized his dream and opened his CrossFit gym. Through his role as a gym owner, he not only assisted people in achieving their overall health and fitness goals but also developed methods to enhance the quality of life and physical freedom of his clients consistently and sustainably.

Determined to provide holistic support to his clients, Coach Bronson embarked on a personal journey of exploring the impact of nutrition on metabolic health and performance. In 2018, he embraced an animal-based nutrition lifestyle, significantly optimizing his well-being. Inspired by the profound effects of combining nutrition and fitness, Bronson developed the F2 Method to radically improve the lives of people across the globe.

Bronson's expertise and passion for health and fitness extend beyond his gym. As an accomplished author, he published the influential book, "The Ultimate Ketogenic Fitness Book: A Complete Guide to Optimizing Keto for a Better Quality of Life." This comprehensive guide has empowered countless people to unlock their full potential by fusing ketogenic principles and fitness practices.

Recognizing the power of personal interaction and tailored guidance, Coach Bronson offers personalized coaching programs and one-on-one consultations. Additionally, he organizes a highly successful life transformation boot camp that caters to people from diverse backgrounds and walks of life.

Bronson's personal health journey began in his late thirties when he found himself struggling with numerous health issues. At that time, he was overweight by seventy pounds, battled with urgent bowels, chronic injuries, and experienced feelings of depression and dissatisfaction with his overall well-being. However, with determination and perseverance, Bronson overcame these obstacles and transformed his life.

Now, at fifty-one, Bronson stands in the prime of his life. He has achieved an impressive level of fitness and possesses a deep-rooted passion for empowering others to learn from his experiences and become the best versions of themselves. With his wealth of knowledge, unwavering dedication, and personal triumphs, Coach Bronson continues to inspire and guide countless others on their journeys toward health, happiness, being body confident.